The Vegan Cookbook for Athletes

Over 100 Plant Based Recipes for High Protein Healthy Nutrition for Athletes with 7 days Meal Plans for increasing Strength and Endurance

By melinda turner

Table of Contents

Introduction
Part 1: Getting Started with Vegan Diet
Chapter 1: Introduction to Vegan Diet
1.1. Purposes behind Following a Plant-Based Diet
1.2. Different Types of Plant-Based Diets
1.3. Benefits of Plant-Based Diet
1.4. Shopping List for Plant-Based Diet
1.5. Nutrient Considerations and Recommendations for Athletes
Part 2: Healthy and Delicious Vegan Recipes
Chapter 2: 100 Vegan Meal Prep Ideas
2.1. Healthy Breakfast Recipes
2.2. Vegan Soups, Salads and Snacks Recipes
2.3. Smoothies and Beverages
2.4. Lunch & Dinner Recipes
2.5. Delicious Vegan Dessert Recipes
Part 3: 7 Day Sample Meal Plans
Chapter 3: Sample Meal Plans to increase Strength and Endurance
3.1. Vegan Sample Meal Plan for Increasing Strength
3.2 Vegan Sample Meal Plan for Increasing Endurance
Conclusion

© **Copyright belinda turner - All rights reserved.**

This document is geared towards providing exact and reliable information in regards to the topic and issue covered. The publication is sold with the idea that the publisher is not required to render accounting, officially permitted, or otherwise, qualified services. If advice is necessary, legal or professional, a practiced individual in the profession should be ordered.

- From a Declaration of Principles which was accepted and approved equally by a Committee of the American Bar Association and a Committee of Publishers and Associations.

In no way is it legal to reproduce, duplicate, or transmit any part of this document in either electronic means or in printed format. Recording of this publication is strictly prohibited and any storage of this document is not allowed unless with written permission from the publisher. All rights reserved.

The information provided herein is stated to be truthful and consistent, in that any liability, in terms of inattention or otherwise, by any usage or abuse of any policies, processes, or directions contained within is the solitary and utter responsibility of the recipient reader. Under no circumstances will any legal responsibility or blame be held against the publisher for any reparation, damages, or monetary loss due to the information herein, either directly or indirectly.

Respective authors own all copyrights not held by the publisher.

The information herein is offered for informational purposes solely, and is universal as so. The presentation of the information is without contract or any type of guarantee assurance. The trademarks that are used are without any consent, and the publication of the trademark is without permission or backing by the trademark owner. All trademarks and brands within this book are for clarifying purposes only and are the owned by the owners themselves, not affiliated with this document.

TABLE OF CONTENTS
INTRODUCTION
PART 1: GETTING STARTED WITH VEGAN DIET
CHAPTER 1: INTRODUCTION TO VEGAN DIET
 1.1. Purposes behind Following a Plant-Based Diet
 1.2. Different Types of Plant-Based Diets
 1.3. Benefits of Plant-Based Diet
 1.4. Shopping List for Plant-Based Diet
 1.5. Nutrient Considerations and Recommendations for Athletes
PART 2: HEALTHY AND DELICIOUS VEGAN RECIPES
CHAPTER 2: 100 VEGAN MEAL PREP IDEAS
2.1. Healthy Breakfast Recipes
2.2. Vegan Soups, Salads and Snacks Recipes
2.3. Smoothies and Beverages
2.4. Lunch & Dinner Recipes

  2.5. Delicious Vegan Dessert Recipes
PART 3: 7 DAY SAMPLE MEAL PLANS
CHAPTER 3: SAMPLE MEAL PLANS TO INCREASE STRENGTH AND ENDURANCE
  3.1. Vegan Sample Meal Plan for Increasing Strength
  3.2 Vegan Sample Meal Plan for Increasing Endurance
CONCLUSION

Introduction

Athletes prefer to adopt vegetarian diets for nutritional, economic, social, political, spiritual/religious and esthetic reasons which may include meat dislike.

While vegetarian diets are quite well-accepted in the global health arena, some coaches and practitioners raise concerns that vegetarian athletes may not get the proper nutrition needed for optimal training and success. In reality, from the various types of vegetarian foods, casual to professional vegetarian athletes can fulfil their energy and nutrient requirements. Around the same time, athletes may reduce their risk of chronic diseases and improve their ability to perform efficiently or recover from extreme exercise.

To ensure optimal efficiency, vegetarian athletes have to consume enough calories and choose foods that are rich in the nutrients of the "red flag," which are either less available in vegetarian foods or less well absorbed from plants compared to animal sources. As with most athletes, vegetarian athletes will benefit from food choices education to improve their productivity and fitness. Please read below if you want to know everything about the vegan diet and how athletes can benefit from the diet and fulfil their nutritional requirements and energy needs from plant-based foods only.

Part 1: Getting Started with Vegan Diet

The Academy of Nutrition and Dietetics says an appropriately prepared vegan diet is safe for all life stages. They also recommend that diets based on plants will offer a range of preventive health benefits. Of course, a poorly designed vegan diet, as with any diet, maybe unsafe or unhealthy.

Such four food classes comprise a healthy vegan diet: 1) legumes, nuts, and seeds; 2) grains; 3) vegetables; and 4) fruits.

Since individual nutrient requirements and energy needs differ by age, level of activity, and health status, this book can only be viewed as a specific guide for a healthy vegan diet. For a personalized collection of guidelines, you can consult a dietitian who is familiar with vegan eating.

Chapter 1: Introduction to Vegan Diet

Veganism has become more and more popular. Many celebrities have turned vegan over the last few years, and a number of vegan items have appeared over supermarkets.

Yet you may be curious as to what this style of eating involves — and what you can and cannot consume on a vegan diet.

In 1944 the word "vegan" was invented by a tiny minority of vegetarians who declared independence from England's Leicester Vegetarian Society to form the Vegan Society.

In addition to refraining from meat, they opted not to consume dairy, eggs or any other items of animal origin, much as vegetarians do.

The word "vegan" was chosen by combining "vegetarian" letters first and last. At the moment, veganism is defined as a way of life which attempts to exclude from food, clothing or any other reason all forms of animal abuse and cruelty.

1.1. Purposes behind Following a Plant-Based Diet

Going vegan is a perfect chance to learn more about health and nutrition. Having your nutrients from plant sources makes more room in your diet for health-promoting choices such as whole grains, berries, nuts, seeds and vegetables, packed full of beneficial fiber, vitamins and minerals.

- **Animal Cruelty**

It is appealing to want to assume that the meat we consume is humane, that our 'food animals' have lived healthy, happy lives and that at the slaughterhouse they have not endured any pain or fear.

Yet the sad fact is, just as we do, all living beings (even those called 'free-range' or 'organic') fear death. All feel the same terror when it comes to slaughter, no matter how they are handled while alive.

The misery of the dairy and egg industry might be less well known than the condition of farmed animals in the factory.

The manufacturing of dairy products requires the death of countless bull calves that are of little benefit to the dairy farmer, as well as the early death of slaughtered cows as their milk production declines.

Likewise, also 'reasonable' or 'free range' eggs in the egg industry include killing the 'unnecessary' male chicks when they are only one day old.

- **Impact on the Environment**

We are all mindful of ways to lead a greener life, from recycling our domestic rubbish to commuting to work. One of the crucial things someone can do to reduce their carbon footprint is to avoid all products of the animals. It goes far beyond the cow-flatulence issue. Processing of meat and dairy products puts a heavy burden on the environment-from the crops and water to sustain the animals, to the transport and other procedures from farm to fork involved. A significant contributor to deforestation, habitat destruction and loss of biodiversity is the large amount of grain feed needed for meat production. Around 5.6 million acres of land in Brazil is used to raise soya beans for livestock in Europe. This land contributes to the production of malnutrition in the developing countries by pushing poor people to cultivate cash crops for livestock feed rather than for themselves. On the other hand, substantially lower crop and water amounts are required to maintain a vegan diet, making the transition to veganism one of the simplest, most friendly and most efficient ways to minimize our impact on the environment.

- **Religious and Spiritual Reasons**

The relation, as it turns out, is nothing new. In traditional Eastern religions including as Hinduism, Buddhism, and Jainism, the virtue of 'ahimsa' is very important, roughly interpreted as 'non-harming'. Supporters of these religions are encouraged to practice vegetarianism or even expected to.

Practically every religion's main values advocate keeping animal products off our tables. All major religions have a principle along the line of "Treat everyone as you want to be treated." None of us wants to become dinner of someone else. Yet most followers of modern religions such as Christianity strongly disagree that animals are subject to such laws. Often, they seek to explain this by saying that animals do not really have souls, or are less valuable than us, or that God has put animals here for us to feed.

Ahimsa refers to all beings since it is believed they all have divine spiritual powers. Harming others means hurting ourselves because we all share the same energy. To put it another way, everything is related - the way we treat animals has significant implications for our society.

Many spiritual individuals see themselves as members of the 'life circle'. They think it is normal and appropriate because other species consume meat, and humans have done so for thousands of years. Yet primitive human beings have no choice but to consume meat for survival, and carnivorous animals do not. This is quite far away from purchasing factory-farmed meat from a supermarket. When we have the option to do otherwise, it can never be acceptable to hurt others.

We all realize in our hearts that it is wrong to hurt other creatures and that all living beings should be respected. Yet some people behave as if spirituality is something abstract, disconnected from our everyday acts. This disconnection helps them to find themselves as spiritual while still eating animal products.

It can be distressing when our convictions and behaviors are not matched. Many people also seek to alter their views to remove this pain without the discomfort of modifying their behavior, for example, by pretending not to care about animal suffering. To practice, veganism means to reject this and to align our actions with our beliefs.

We are grateful to be living in a community where healthy and nutritious food can be enjoyed without hurting or abusing animals. Ultimately, a lifestyle that causes minimal harm to animals' benefits everyone and all else on the planet, as everything is related. Whether your perspective is rational, spiritual or a bit of both, being vegan just makes sense.

Bottom Line

The happy news is we can do something to change it. We may choose to support these animals and our environment whenever we buy or order food in a restaurant. We stand up for farmed animals everywhere every time we make the transition from an animal product to a vegan one. Going vegan is simpler than ever before with veganism gradually becoming popular as more and more people of all backgrounds, ages and races are discovering the benefits of living this way.

1.2. Different Types of Plant-Based Diets

- **Vegan Whole-Food Diet**

A diet focused on a broad range of foods from whole plants including vegetables, fruits, whole grains, nuts, legumes and seeds.

- **80|10|10 Diet**

This diet is a vegan raw-food diet that limits to fat-rich plants like nuts and avocados and mainly depends on soft greens and raw fruits instead. It is also referred to as low-fat, vegan raw-food diet or fruit diet.

- **Vegan Raw-food Diet**

A vegan diet focused on raw fruits, berries, seeds, nuts or plant products that are cooked under 118 ° F (48 ° C).

- **Raw till 4 P.m. Diet**

This low-fat vegan diet is a combination of the starch and 80|10|10 diet. Raw foods are eaten for dinner before 4 p.m., with the choice of a cooked plant-based meal.

- **The Starch Diet**

A high-carb, low-fat vegan diet closely related to that of the 80|10|10 but focused on cooked starch food such as rice, corn and potatoes instead of fruit.

- **The Thrive Diet**

This diet is a vegan raw-food diet. Followers consume whole plant-based, raw or moderately cooked foods at low temperatures.

- **Vegan Junk-Food Diet**

This vegan diet lacks foods from whole plants and heavily relies on mock meats and cheeses, vegan desserts and other overly processed vegan foods.

A vegan diet can be followed in several ways, but scientific research rarely differentiates between the different types.

1.3. Benefits of Plant-Based Diet

Rich in vegetables, fruits, legumes and nuts and seeds, a plant-based diet is a perfect way to maintain good health. These foods are rich in vitamins, fibers and minerals, cholesterol-free and low in saturated fat and calories.

Consuming a variety of these foods gives the body all the protein, calcium and other vital nutrients that it requires. Including a reliable vitamin B12 source into your diet is also critical. With a vitamin supplement or fortified food, like vitamin B12-fortified breakfast cereals, plant milk, and nutritional yeast, you can easily satisfy your vitamin B12 needs.

1) **Plant-Based Diet as Medicine**

Research indicates that plant-based diets are low-risk and cost-effective treatments that may decrease body mass index, blood pressure, HbA1C, and levels of cholesterol.

These can also reduce the amount of medicines required to treat chronic diseases and decrease the mortality rates for ischemic heart disease.

A plant-based diet should be prescribed to all patients by doctors, particularly those with high blood pressure, diabetes, cardiovascular disease, or obesity.

- **Lowers Blood Sugar Levels**

Plant diets prevent, treat and cure type II diabetes. Plant-based diets lower body weight, boost insulin production and increase the capacity of beta-cells to control blood sugar, which reverses symptoms of type II diabetes.

- **Reduce Cardiovascular Risk by Reducing Cholesterol Level**

Those who consume a diet based on plants have a lower chance of dying from heart disease compared with non-vegetarians. It has been proven that plant-based diets prevent and cure heart disease, lower blood pressure and improve cholesterol.

- **Lower the Risk of Contracting other Cancers, such as Colon Cancer**

Avoiding animal products and high-fat foods, as well as eating plant-based foods can reduce the risk of having certain cancers.

- **Brain Health**

Trans fat and saturated fat – found in meat, dairy products and fried foods – may significantly raise the risk of Alzheimer's disease and other cognitive conditions.

A plant-based diet prevents these foods and is high in antioxidants, folate, and vitamin E, which can be healthy.

2) Vegan Diet for Weight Loss

You might have considered attempting a plant-based diet if you are looking to lose any pounds. Vegans consume no meat, fish, eggs or dairy products. They eat foods like fresh vegetables and fruits, legumes and beans and even plant-based milk, other non-dairy foods, and meat substitutes.

While some people adopt the lifestyle of a vegan because of animal rights and other issues, but the diet has certain health benefits itself. Going vegan can also aid in substantial weight loss according to recent studies.

Exactly how? More work is required, but it is assumed that switching to veganism will lead to a reduction in the amount of rich-calorie foods you eat. With a vegan diet, you replace such foods with high-fiber substitutes that have fewer calories and keep you fuller for longer.

3) Benefits for Athletes

How, exactly, does going vegan give the athletes (amateurs and pros alike) a competitive edge? The answer is given below:

- Even athletes are at risk for cardiac disease: 44 per cent of professional cyclists and runners had coronary plaques, shown in one study. A plant-based diet keeps the hearts of athletes healthy by removing the plaque, lowering blood pressure and cholesterol, and weight loss.
- Consumption of meat and high levels of cholesterol exacerbate inflammation, leading to pain and impairing athletic performance and recovery. Studies show a diet focused on plants can have an anti-inflammatory effect.
- A low-saturated, cholesterol-free plant-based diet helps increase blood thickness or viscosity. That helps the muscles to reach more oxygen, improving the performance of athletes.
- Plant-based diets maximize arterial strength and diameter, resulting in increased blood flow. One analysis revealed that even a single high-fat meal, including McMuffins sausage and egg, has had several hours of impaired arterial function.

- People consuming a plant-based diet get much more antioxidants opposed to meat-eaters, which help to neutralize free radicals; Free radicals contribute to weakness in the muscles, reduced athletic efficiency and impaired recovery.
- Vegetable diets usually high in fiber and low in fat can reduce body fat. Reduced body fat is correlated with improved aerobic capacity — or the ability to sustain exercise using oxygen. Research indicates that plant-based dietary athletes increase their VO2 max — the maximum amount of oxygen they can use during vigorous exercise — contributing to increased stamina.

1.4. Shopping List for Plant-Based Diet

- **Vegetables and Fruits**

Both are perfect foods for increasing your nutrient intake. In particular, leafy greens like bok choy, kale, spinach, mustard greens and watercress are rich in calcium and iron.

- **Calcium-Fortified Plant Yoghurts and Milk**

These help vegans meet their recommended levels of calcium in the diet. If possible, opt for varieties often fortified with vitamins B12 and D.

- **The Flax, Hemp and Chia Seeds**

Hemp, chia and flaxseeds, in particular, contain a decent amount of protein and beneficial omega-3 fatty acids

- **Butters Nuts and Nuts**

Especially unroasted and unbalanced varieties are good sources of iron, magnesium, fiber, selenium, zinc and vitamin E.

- **Legumes**

Foods like beans, peas and lentils are excellent sources of various nutrients and beneficial compounds for plants. Sprinkling, fermentation and proper cooking will improve nutrient absorption.

- **Tofu and other Alternatives for Minimally Processed Meat**

For several recipes, these provide a versatile protein-rich alternative to meat, poultry, fish and eggs.

- **Ground, Fermented Plant Foods**

Ezekiel's pasta, natto, Misco, tempeh, sauerkraut, pickles, kimchi, and kombucha also contain vitamin K2 and probiotics. Fermentation and sprouting can also help increase the mineral absorption.

- **Whole Wheat and Pseudo Cereals**

They are a perfect source of complex carbohydrates, nutrients, magnesium, B-vitamins and minerals. Spelt, teff, amaranth and quinoa are especially protein-rich choices.

- **Nutritional Yeast**

It is a simple way to increase vegan dishes protein content and add an interesting cheesy flavor. Pick varieties that are fortified with vitamin B12 wherever possible.

- **Algae**

Spirulina and chlorella are healthy, complete protein sources. Other varieties are major iodine sources.

Bottom Line:

Such minimally processed plant foods constitute perfect additions to every vegan pantry or refrigerator.

1.5. Nutrient Considerations and Recommendations for Athletes

While it is not completely important to grab the calculator and find out your optimal daily calorie intake, and how to split this figure into fat, carbohydrates and protein components, but for professional athletes, it is worth it.

With the disclaimer that it is just an approximation due to factors like body mass, level of fitness and metabolic rate, you can use the formula below to calculate your daily caloric needs. In a laboratory, your caloric requirements can be calculated through indirect or direct calorimetry for a more accurate assessment.

First, you need to know your age, height, and weight to measure your Basal Metabolic Rate (BMR). BMR calculates how many calories you need to sustain life if you are entirely immobile; that is, it is the strength you just need to be alive!

BMR of Women
BMR of Men

Next step is to use the formula of Harris-Benedict to multiply the BMR with the correct factor of physical activity. When you happen to be

Sedentary (limited or no workout)	1.2×BMR = Calories required per day
Lightly engaged (light sport/ exercise for 1 or 3 days a week)	1.375×BMR = Calories required per day
Moderately engaged (3 or 5 days a week mild exercise / sport)	1.55×BMR = Calories required per day
Quite active (hard workout / sport 6 or 7 days/week)	1.725×BMR = Calories required per day
Highly active (very tough exercise/sports or physical activity or 2 times training)	1.9×BMR = Calories required per day

So, the problem is: Is it possible to get all the calories you required from plants? Be assured you can, with ease. For example, in his book "Food for Fitness", a renowned cycling coach, Chris Carmichael recommends that athletes obtain about 65% of the caloric needs from carbohydrates, 22% from fats and 13% from proteins. The numbers are not extraordinary, and can be quickly achieved consuming a diet based on plant.

Calculate your Daily Calorie Intake

Let us consider the example and work through the equations of nutrition for you to get an understanding of how to plan your standard day of vegan diet to fulfil your unique nutritional requirements.

Example: Hailey Training for the Marathon

First, let us assume a woman, weight: 130 pounds, Height: 5'2 inches, Age: 26 years, who is preparing for a marathon, and thus exercising 4-5 days a week.

Her BMR is:

655 + (pounds of weight × 4.35) + (inches of height × 4.7) - (years of age × 4.7)

= 655 + (130 × 4.35) + (62 x 4.7) - (26 x 4.7)

= Calories 1,390 per day

As she trains for a marathon and runs 4 to 5 days a week, it is determined that she is "moderately active" using the parameters from above, which means that 1.55 is her activity factor.

So, if we substitute this value in the equation of Harris-Benedict, we will get:

1.390 x 1.55 calories = 2.154 calories required per day. (Note: this is only an average. She will eat more on hard training days to support the exercise and she will usually eat much less than the amount on break or moderate training days.)

Splitting her total of roughly 2,150 calories/day into the nutrient ratios we get:

1. Carbohydrates (65%): 1,398 calories = 65%×2150. Since the carbohydrate content is 4 calories/gram, this amounts to 1,398÷4 = 349.38 (about 350) grams of carbohydrates each day.
2. Protein (13%): 13%×2150, = 280 calories. Since there are 4 calories/gram of carbohydrate, this results in 280÷4 = 69.88 (about 70) grams of protein/day.
3. Fat (22%) = 473 calories: 23%×2150. Since there are 9 calories/gram of fat, this amounts to 473÷9 = 52.5 (about 53) grams of fat/day.

Other Nutrient Recommendations:

Nutrients	Sources
Healthy Fats	Nuts, nut butters, seeds, avocado, olive oil, olives, flaxseed, granola, coconut, and muesli cereals, plant-based oils including grape seed, canola, hazelnut, pumpkin seed, sesame seed and hemp oils.
Protein	Yoghurt, milk, cottage cheese, eggs, peas, beans lentils, tempeh, edamame, tofu, nuts, seeds, soy products, nut butters (including peanut), soymilk and other plant-based milks. Other sources: grains, breads, starchy vegetables, rice, oatmeal, quinoa.
Omega-3 Fatty Acids	Flax, camelina, walnuts chia, hemp seed, walnut, canola, and hemp oils.
Zinc	Beans, lentils, peas, edamame, seeds, nuts, whole & fortified grains including breads, most vegetables, rice, breakfast cereal, quinoa and hard cheeses.
Iron	Lentils, peas, beans, edamame, seeds, nuts, whole & fortified grains including breads, most vegetables, quinoa, rice, breakfast cereal. Absorption strengthened by consumption with vitamin C sources: Berries, citrus fruits, melon, tomatoes, peppers, broccoli,

	potatoes and kale.
Calcium	Excellent bioavailability (> 50%): Bok choy, Chinese cabbage, kale, collards, turnip greens, okra, texturized vegetable proteins, blackstrap molasses. Average bioavailability (~30%): Yogurt, milk, cheese, fortified orange juice, calcium-set tofu. Lower bioavailability: Most nuts, fortified soymilk, seeds legumes and fortified orange juice.
Vitamin D	Eggs from hens exposed to sunlight or fed vitamin D, fatty fish, fruit juice, margarine, vitamin D-fortified breakfast cereals and plant-based milk. Arms legs and torso exposure, 2 to 3 times a week, near solar noon for 25-50% of the time it would take for a mild sunburn to develop.
Vitamin B-12	Soymilk & plant-based milks, breakfast cereals, nutritional yeast and B-12 fortified meat analogues
Iodine	Fish, Iodized salt, seafood, dairy products seaweed and some commercial-breads.

Part 2: Healthy and Delicious Vegan Recipes

Vegan recipes can often sound a little complicated and laborious. That is why below is a list of ideas for vegan breakfast, lunch and dinner that are not just tasty but quick to make. If you are just starting on a vegan diet, or trying it out for a few weeks only, or you are a plant-based expert, these 100 delicious recipes are a perfect way to figure out your weekly meal plan.

Chapter 2: 100 Vegan Meal Prep Ideas

It takes a little expertise to recreate traditional oil-loaded classics like French fries, pesto, quesadillas, fried rice, hash browns, tacos, desserts, salads, and salad dressings without the added fat.

But do not worry: These enticing recipes use simple cooking methods such as steaming, baking, breading, pan-toasting, roasting and sautéing so you can skip the oil without skimping on flavor.

You will never run out of snacks, breakfast, lunch, dinner or dessert options with too many vegan meal planning recipes to choose from!

2.1. Healthy Breakfast Recipes

Preparing your breakfasts ahead is a perfect way to alleviate your morning tension and begin your day off on a safe note. All these vegan meal planning breakfast recipes are refrigerator-friendly, and some are fridge-friendly too.

1) Overnight Oats with Fruits on Bottom

Overnight oats with fruits on the bottom do not need to cook, and are ideal for meal preparations! Just five basic ingredients and meal is ready within 10 minutes.

Calories: 343 kcal| Serves: 1| Prep Time: 10 mins| Total Time: 10 mins

Ingredients:
- Frozen thawed fruit: 1 cup
- Chia seeds: 1 tablespoon
- Almond milk: 3/4 cup
- Maple syrup: 1 teaspoon
- Rolled oats: 1/2 cup

Directions:
1. Place the frozen fruit thawed at the bottom of a container (at least 12.5 oz; 1 pint works too). Use a spatula and mash to make a puree.
2. Add maple syrup, almond milk, rolled oats, and chia seeds. No need to mix, just place the lid on and refrigerate overnight.
3. You can store it for four days. Serve cold.

2) Scrambled Tofu

Prepare Time: 5-6 minutes| Cooking Time: 10 minutes| Total Time: 15 minutes| Serves: 2

Ingredients:
- Firm tofu: (225 g) 8 ounces
- Salt: 1/4 teaspoon
- Turmeric powder: 1/4 teaspoon
- Black pepper: 1/8 teaspoon

Directions:
1. Cut the cubes of tofu and crumble it into small chunks using a fork.
2. Take a saucepan and add some oil, add the tofu when the oil gets hot, and all other ingredients (turmeric powder, and ground black pepper and salt). Mix it well, and cook 5-10 minutes over medium-high heat. Occasionally stir.
3. Serve immediately with fresh vegetables, vegan bacon or vegan sausages as part of a vegan brunch. It can also be eaten with vegan pancakes and with coffee or tea.
4. Keep the leftovers in the refrigerator in an airtight jar for up to 1 week. You can also preserve and prepare the tofu before cooking for up to 5 months.

3) Baked Oatmeal Muffins

Baked oatmeal muffins are a delicious breakfast meal or snack on the go. These are easily made gluten-free and vegan, freezer-friendly, and are customizable with seven different combinations of flavor, so you will never get bored!

Prep Time: 10 minutes | Time to Cook: 25 minutes | Total time: 35 minutes | Serves: 8 | 132 Kcal Calories

Ingredients:
Basic Recipe:
- Simple traditional oats: 1 1/2 cups
- Cinnamon: 1/2 teaspoon
- Baking Powder: 1 teaspoon
- Egg: 1 Large
- Maple syrup: 1/4 cup
- Milk: 1 cup

Blueberry and Almonds:
- Traditional oats: 1 1/2 cups
- Cinnamon: 1/2 teaspoon
- Baking Powder: 1/2 teaspoon
- Egg: 1 large
- Honey or maple syrup: 1/4 cup
- Any kind of milk: 1 cup
- Frozen blueberries: 1 cup
- Chopped Almonds: 1/4 cup

Directions:
1. Preheat oven to 350°F. Place a silicone or parchment lining muffin sheet, or spray generously with oil.
2. Use a large bowl and mix all the ingredients (preferably with a spout). Spoon into the liners of the prepared muffins. Try to get oat mixture and liquid divided evenly among all liners.
3. Bake 20-25 minutes, until golden and not jiggling any more.
4. Before serving cool it completely.

4) Chocolate Pudding with Chia

Made with only 6-ingredients this pudding is creamy, naturally sweetened and thick. Nutrient filled and good for breakfast, snack or dessert!

Prep Time: 3 hours| Total Time: 3 hours | Servings: 4 cups

Ingredients:
- Powdered cocoa or unsweetened raw cocoa: 1/4 cup:
- Maple syrup: 3 -5 tablespoon
- Ground cinnamon: 1/2 teaspoon
- 1 Pinch salt
- Vanilla extract: 1/2 teaspoon.
- Unsweetened Almond milk: 1 1/2 cups
- Chia Seeds: 1/2 cup

Instructions:
1. Add cacao powder, maple syrup, salt, ground cinnamon, and vanilla to a small or medium mixing bowl and whisk. Then add almond milk at once while whisking until it forms a paste. Add remaining milk and blend until smooth.

2. Next put chia seeds in it and blend once again. Then cover and rest aside for at least 3-5 hours or overnight (until desired consistency is achieved). Give the mixture an extra stir/whisk after 30-45 minutes in the refrigerator.
3. Store the leftovers in the refrigerator for 4-5 days. Serve with toppings of your choice such as fruit, granola or whipped cream made from coconut.

5) Vegan Miso Biscuits and Green Onions

Serves: 8 cookies

Ingredients:
- Whole pastry wheat flour: 2 cups
- Aluminum-free baking powder: 1 spoonful
- Baking soda: ½ Teaspoon
- Nutritional yeast: 1 tablespoon
- Fine sea salt: 3/4 teaspoon
- Vegan butter: 3/4 cup
- Green onions, finely sliced: 2 tablespoons plus extra for garnish
- Unsweetened non-dairy milk, divided: 2/3 cup + 2 tablespoon
- Apple cider vinegar: 1/2 teaspoon
- Light miso: 1 tablespoon
- Pure maple syrup: 1/2 teaspoon

Instructions:
1. Oven preheated to 425 F. Line a parchment baking sheet and set aside.
2. Whisk the flour, baking powder, nutritional yeast, baking soda, salt and green onions in a large bowl.
3. Place a box grater right over the flour mixture in the large tub. Grate the vegan butter into the bowl, quickly. For 10 minutes, place the bowl in the freezer.
4. Whisk 2/3 cup of the non-dairy milk, apple cider vinegar, and miso together in a small bowl.
5. Take the grated butter and flour mixture out of the freezer. Quickly mix the butter into the flour with your hands until you have a coarse mixture. It should be pretty firm. Once the butter has been added (you may want to see some tiny grated bits), add flour and butter to the non-dairy milk mixture.
6. Stir the biscuit batter quickly and fold until it all starts to get together and is evenly hydrated. Flour a surface and pour the dough out.
7. Form the biscuit dough into an even-thick rectangle, around an inch and a half. Cut the dough into just eight squares. Carry the biscuits carefully onto the baking sheet. Put the baking sheet in the freezer for 10 or 12 minutes, to make the batter firm.
8. When the biscuits are retrieved, whisk the remaining non-dairy milk and maple syrup together. Brush the mixture over the cookies. Sprinkle on top with extra sliced green onions, black pepper and flaky sea salt, if you want.

9. Slide the vegan biscuits into the oven and bake for 13-17 minutes or until golden brown on the edges and the biscuits are puffed up. Let the biscuits cool down before eating.

6) Yogurt and Fruit Tart

Vegan Fruit and Yogurt Breakfast Tart make every occasion a sweet, non-dairy breakfast treat. Customize your balanced tartar with seasonal fruit of your choice.

Prepare Time: 14-15 minutes | Cook Time: 15 minutes| Yield: 8 servings

Ingredients:

Crust:
- Traditional oats: 1 1/2 cups
- Chopped nuts and seeds like almonds, pistachios, hazelnuts, walnuts, grains of pumpkin, sesame seeds: 1 cup
- Coconut oil, melt if solid: 1/4 cup
- Brown sugar: 2 tablespoons
- Vanilla extract: 1 teaspoon

Filling and Topping:
- Container Vanilla So Delicious Coconut Milk Yogurt Alternative: 24-Ounce
- Thinly sliced starfruit: 1 big or 2 smalls
- Strawberries: 2-3 Sliced
- Mandarin orange slices: ½ cup
- Blueberries: 1/2 cup
- Thinly sliced mango or papaya and cup into a small heart with a small cutter: 1
- Sliced and peeled kiwi: 1
- Bananas: 1/2
- Raspberries: Around 10

Directions:
1. Preheat oven to 350 F.
2. In a bowl, combine the oats, seeds and nuts, coconut oil, sugar and vanilla until all is well coated.
3. Place the mixture into a greased 10-12 "tart pan with a removable bottom (or pie plate) and use a measuring cup to help spread the granola uniformly around the pan and up the sides.
4. Bake for about 13 or 15 minutes, until lightly golden. Let it cool. If you want to, you can make the crust ahead and fill it just before serving the next morning.
5. Spread the yoghurt uniformly over the crust of cooled granola.
6. Put the strawberries along with the starfruit slices starting at the outer edge. Add slices of orange mandarin into the gaps between them and then make a circle of blueberries around it. Follow with the raspberries and mango hearts.
7. Arrange half kiwi moons next, and then fill in with banana slices, raspberries and blueberry in the middle.

8. Serve straight away for best results. Remove the edges of the tart pan, so it becomes easy to slice the tart. Use a sharp knife to cut the slices through the crust and ease them out with a pie server.

7) Jelly Chia Pudding and Peanut Butter

This peanut butter jelly chia pudding is sweetened naturally and can be quickly prepared with 7 simple ingredients. A breakfast which is healthy, delicious and satisfying!

Ingredients:
- Fresh or frozen blueberries: 1 tablespoon
- Orange juice: 1 tablespoon
- Chia seeds: 1 tablespoon
- Unsweetened almond milk: 1 cup
- Coconut milk: 1/2 cup
- Vanilla: 1 teaspoon
- Maple syrup: 1-2 tablespoons
- Salted natural peanut butter: 3 tablespoons, plus more for serving):
- Chia seeds: 1/3 cup
- For toppings: fresh blueberries

Directions:
1. Add the orange juice and blueberries to a saucepan or skillet. Cook over low-medium heat until bubbles appear. Lower to medium heat then cook for two minutes-stirring periodically. Turn off the heat, and add the seeds of chia. Stir to mix.
2. Divide the mixture between three small serving bowls, and put to chill in the refrigerator.
3. Meanwhile, add the coconut and almond milk together with maple syrup, peanut butter, and vanilla (optional) to a blender. Mix on high speed to combine thoroughly. For sweetness add maple syrup or for saltiness add peanut butter to change flavors as required.
4. Put chia seeds in a blender and blend, but do not to blend enough as you need the seeds left whole.
5. Put the mixture into a jar and set it in the refrigerator to chill.
6. Wait 10-12 minutes to cool down the compote. Then remove from the fridge the compote and pudding. Stir the pudding to scatter the chia seeds, then separate the pudding, layering on top of the compote into three serving bowls.
7. Cover the bowls and set for 2-3 hours in the refrigerator, or until desired consistency of pudding is achieved.
8. When serving, top with more blueberries and peanut butter.

8) Chocolate Chip – Oatmeal Pancake

A new and improved version of the famous chocolate chip oatmeal pancakes, this time rendered gluten-free, vegan and only 30 minutes needed!
Prepare Time: 14 minutes| Cook Time: 8 minutes| Total Time: 23 minutes| Serves: 2
Ingredients:

- Flax eggs: 1 batch
- Ripe medium banana: (1 mashed banana yield ~ 1/2 cup)
- Baking Powder: 1 Tsp
- Salt: 1 pinch
- Vanilla extract: 1/2 teaspoon (optional)
- Almond butter: 1 tablespoon
- Avocado oil: 1 tablespoon
- Unsweetened almond milk: 1/3 tablespoon
- Rolled gluten-free oats: 1/2 cup
- Almond meal: 2 tablespoons
- Mixture of gluten-free flour: 1/4 cup
- Non-milky half-sweet chocolate chips: 3 tablespoons or more for topping
- 1 teaspoon agave or maple syrup

Directions:
1. Prepare flax eggs in a wide bowl by mixing flaxseed meal with water and letting it sit for 3-5 minutes.
2. Mash your very ripe banana, add baking powder and mash again.
3. Add sugar, salt, vanilla, almonds butter and pour in almond milk and mix well.
4. Mix oats, almond meal, and gluten-free flour until combined.
5. Sprinkle in chocolate chips then gently fold. Let the oven preheat to medium-low heat and let it rest for 5 minutes. You want it hot but not too hot or the pancakes will burn-between 300-325 degrees.
6. To make a pancake shape, scoop 1/4 cup measurements onto the lightly-greased griddle and spread gently. Bake each side for 3-4 minutes, until golden brown. You will know when bubbles grow on top; they are ready to turn.
7. Serve as is or with a quick maple syrup drizzle, and a few extra chocolate chips. Leftovers will again heat up well in the microwave.

9) Vegan Apple Pie Cake with Cinnamon Custard

Quick, soft and light apple cake, serve with custard made of smooth organic vanilla.
Cook Time: 40 Minutes | Preparation Time: 15 Minutes| Full Time 55 Minutes | Servings: 9 Slices | Calories: 205kcal

Wet Ingredients:
- Almond milk: 1 cup (244 g)
- Applesauce or non-milk yoghurt: 2 tablespoons
- Cider vinegar: 1 teaspoon
- Sugar: 1/3 cup (66.67 g)
- Vanilla: 1 teaspoon
- Almond extract: Few drops (optional)

Dry Ingredients:
- Flour: 187.5 g (1.5 to 1.75 cups)
- Baking powder: 2 tablespoons
- Baking soda: 1/4 teaspoon

- Pumpkin or cinnamon pie spice: 1/2 teaspoon
- Salt: 1/2 teaspoon
- Apple: 1, small and chopped
- Maple syrup: 1 tablespoon
- Coconut sugar: 1.5 Tablespoon

Custard Ingredients:
- 1 cup (236.59 ml) + 1/4 cup non-dairy milk
- Sugar or sweetener: 2 tablespoons
- Vanilla extract: 1/2 teaspoon
- Almond extract: 2 drops
- Salt: a pinch
- Potato starch or corn starch: 1 tablespoon
- Cinnamon 1/8 tsp
- Turmeric 1/8 teaspoon (optional)

Directions:
1. Line a pan with a parchment hanging at the bottom. Set the oven and preheat up to 350 degree F (176 C). Blend the wet ingredients for the cake in a bowl, until the sugar is thoroughly mixed.
2. Add 1 1/2 cup flour, baking powder, baking soda, salt and cinnamon.
3. Fold into the wet mixture till combined. To make the batter slightly thick, add more flour if required, 1 tablespoon at a time.
4. Drizzle the maple over the chopped apple in another bowl, and toss to coat. Add apple and fold into batter.
5. Pour into the lined pan and even it out. Sprinkle sugar with coconut over a batter
6. Bake for 35 to 45 mins in the oven at 350 degrees F. Cool for 10 minutes and then remove from pan. Cool before slicing. Store for the day at your counter, refrigerated for up to 7 days, freeze (slices) for up to one month
7. Make cupcakes/muffins: Bake for standard size muffins for 22 to 24 mins.

Custard:
1. Mix the sugar, vanilla extract, almond extract and non-dairy milk in a saucepan and boil over medium heat. Add cinnamon or other flavors, as appropriate. For color, add a pinch of turmeric.
2. In 1/4 cup of non-dairy milk, mix the starch, then add to the boiling milk. Bring to a strong boil, and then instantly turn off the heat. Custard is getting thickened as it cools. (Serve slices of apple cake sliced with custard.

10) Avocado Tofu Toast

Prep Time: 10-12 mins| Cook Time: 30 mins| Total Time: 50 mins| Yield: 4 servings

Ingredients:
- Firm tofu block: 1 (12-ounce), pressed and drained
- Coconut oil spray
- Avocado: 1 sliced

- Garlic powder: 1/2 teaspoon
- Freshly ground black pepper.
- Red pepper flakes: a pinch
- For serving: thinly cut radishes, sprouts and hard-boiled chopped egg.

Instructions:
1. Set your oven to 425 degrees F and preheat it. Use a baking tray and covert it with parchment paper.
2. Split the block of tofu in half, creating two blocks of about 3/4-inch wide.
3. Then again split the blocks in half, creating 4 triangular blocks of "tofu toast" this time through the middle.
4. Place the tofu onto the baking paper in a single layer. Sprinkle oil on top of the tofu and bake for about 20 minutes until crispy golden and bubbling on top.
5. Take out the tofu from the oven, turn each slice over and sprinkle with oil.
6. Put the tofu back in the oven and cook for another 10 minutes. Rest aside for 5 to 10 minutes to cool.
7. Slather the tofu toast with the garlic powder and sliced avocado to serve. Sprinkle some red pepper, black pepper flakes and layer on radishes, sprouts and hard-boiled egg.

11) Cinnamon Butter and Fig Toast

Active Time: 5 minutes | Total Cooking Time: 5 minutes| Yield: 8 servings

Ingredients:
- Cinnamon Butter
- Plant-based butter: ¼ cup (both avocado oil or coconut oil work)
- Vanilla extract: ¼ teaspoon
- Cinnamon: ½ teaspoon
- Maple syrup: 2 tablespoons
- Cardamom: 1/4 teaspoon (optional)
- Breakfast Fig Toast
- Sourdough bread: 8 slices
- 8–10 fresh figs, sliced into rounds
- Roasted and crushed pistachios
- Flaky sea salt
- Finely chopped fresh mint

Instructions:
1. Mix all the ingredients together for the preparation of cinnamon butter in a sealable container. Taste the seasonings and adjust accordingly. Cover it on and place it in the fridge, ready for use.
2. Preparing the fig toast: Toast the bread until it becomes as crispy golden as you like. Spread the cinnamon butter you made, about 1/2 tablespoon over each slice of toast. Top with pistachios, sliced figs, mint and salt as desired.

12) Sweet Potato Bowl

Prep Time: 5 minutes| Cooking Time: 1 hour 20 minutes| Total Time: 1 hour 25 minutes| Servings: 2|Calories: 356kcal

Ingredients:
- Sweet potato: 1 large or 2 smalls
- Optional: honey OR half of a small, slightly ripe mashed banana for sweetness
- Cinnamon, to taste
- Raisins: 2 tablespoons
- Chopped nuts: 2 tablespoons
- Almond butter: 2 tablespoons

Instructions:
1. Set the oven temperature to 375 degree C and preheat it. Wash, and dry the sweet potato(s) lightly. Use a fork to poke it several times, and cover in aluminum foil.
2. Bake sweet potato for about 70-80 minutes if large, or for about 60-65 minutes if using 2 smalls, until a fork can easily perforate the whole sweet potato. Let cool for a minimum of five minutes before peeling.
3. Peel the cooled sweet potato and mash lightly. Add honey and cinnamon for sweetness (or half mashed banana).
4. Where desired, top with chopped nuts and raisins and drizzle some almond butter over it.

13)   Vegan Almond Granola

This simple granola recipe is all-purpose: Mix it for breakfast with yoghurt, munch on it alone as an office snack or spoon it over vanilla ice cream and cooked dessert fruit.

Calories: 279 kcal| Yield: 12| Prep Time: 5 mins| Cook Time: 55 mins| Total Time: 1 hour

Ingredients:
- Light brown sugar: 1/2 cup
- Canola oil: 1/4 cup
- Vanilla extract: 1 teaspoon
- Kosher salt: 1 teaspoon
- Old-fashioned oats: 4 cups
- Almonds: 1 cup
- Sunflower seeds: 1/2 cup

Instructions:
1. Preheat your oven to 350 degree F. Attach two baking sheets with non-stick foil. Whisk the butter, brown sugar, vanilla and salt together in a large bowl.
2. Add the almonds, oats and sunflower seeds and toss, ensuring oats and nuts are well coated. Split the mixture into the prepared pans. Now, bake for 20 to 25 minutes, tossing once, until crisp and golden brown. Rest aside to cool completely.
3. Granola can be preserved for up to 2 weeks, at room temperature.

14)   Gingerbread Scones with Glaze of Vanilla Bean

Healthier gingerbread scones glazed with vanilla bean, made from wholesome ingredients like wheat pastry flour, coconut sugar and coconut oil!

Preparation Time: 13 mins| Cooking Time: 16 mins| Total Time: 31 mins| Serves: 8

Ingredients:
- Flax egg: 1
- Whole-wheat pastry flour: 2 cups
- Coconut sugar: 1/3 cup
- Baking powder: 1 tablespoon
- Ginger: 1 teaspoon
- Cinnamon: ½ teaspoon
- Cloves: ¼ teaspoon
- Sea salt: ¼ teaspoon
- Almond milk, unsweetened: ½ cup + 2 tablespoon
- Molasses: 1/3 cup
- Coconut oil: 5 tablespoons in a hardened form

For the Glaze:
- ½ vanilla bean
- Powdered sugar: ¾ cup
- Almond milk, unsweetened: 1 tablespoon

Instructions:
1. Preheat the oven to 400 ° C. Prepare a parchment-papered baking dish.
2. Make the flax egg in a small/medium dish. Let it rest for 5 minutes.
3. First, put all your dry ingredients in a large cup, and whisk together.
4. Then add the molasses and almond milk in it. Whisk to blend thoroughly. It takes one minute, or two! Rest aside. Stir the coconut oil in dry ingredients. Cut the coconut oil into the mixture using a pastry cutter or a fork until the coconut oil is the side of the peas or something like that (see image).
5. Next, add your wet ingredients into the dry slowly. Mix until just blended (beware of not over-mixing). A little flour will always be on the bottom of the pot, which is perfect.
6. Place the scone batter on the prepared baking sheet. Shape the batter into a circle of around 7–8 inches.
7. Use a sharp knife and cut eight triangles of equal size.
8. Bake for 14 minutes in the oven.
9. Cut the scones again after the 14 minutes (where you cut earlier) and pull them apart, so the sides have time to bake.
10. Bake another 2-4 minutes (total 16-18) or until golden brown, and cooked through. Cool it for 10 minutes.
11. Put and whisk all the ingredients in a bowl to create the glaze. Drizzle the glaze on top of the scones. For freshness keep scones completely covered.

15) Mushroom Bacon Toast with Hummus

A gluten-free, plant-based breakfast meal that will change the way you think of breakfast!

Preparation Time: 5 minutes | Cooking Time: 30 minutes| Total Time: 35 minutes| Yield: 5

Ingredients:

For the Smoky Bacon:
- Finely chopped mushrooms: 1 1/4 cup or 6 ounces
- Olive oil to drizzle
- Kosher salt and pepper to taste
- Smoked paprika: 1/2 teaspoon OR liquid smoke: 1 teaspoon
- Garlic or onion powder: 1/8 teaspoon
- Coconut sugar or maple syrup: 1 teaspoon

For the breakfast toast:
- Whole grain bread, gluten-free: 4-5 pieces
- 1/2 c + plain Hummus or garlic hummus
- Grape or cherry tomatoes
- Chopped Herbs (fresh parsley or basil)
- Kosher salt and pepper
- Olive oil to drizzle

Other toppings (optional):
- Nutritional yeast "for Cheesy" taste
- Large sea salt flakes
- Red pepper flakes, crushed
- Black pepper or peppercorns, crushed

Instructions:

For smoky mushroom bacon:
1. Set the oven to 375 F and preheat it. Take the parchment paper and line it on a baking sheet, or spray the sheet pan with oil.
2. Cut the mushrooms finely into small chunks and put in a single layer on a sheet. On top of the mushrooms drizzle one teaspoon of olive oil and season with optional kosher salt and pepper.
3. Bake the mushroom for 12-15 minutes. Remove the mushrooms from the oven after 12-15 minutes, and gently turn over mushrooms. Return the mushrooms to the oven, and continue to bake for about 12-15 minutes until crispy and browned.
4. After removing from the oven put the mushrooms in a bowl and drain off the oil. Then toss with maple syrup, coconut sugar, garlic or onion powder, liquid smoke (optional), and smoked paprika. Return to the oven to caramelize the mushrooms for another 5 minutes.
5. Rest aside to top with toast for breakfast later.

Make Toast for your Breakfast:
1. Prepare a sheet pan with tomatoes and toast, before returning the mushrooms to the oven for the second time. Oil the pan and put the toast on it and the tomatoes on a different pan. The tomatoes and toast pan is placed on top or

bottom rack. Bake for 10 minutes or until the tomatoes go blistering and softening and the toasts are browned.
2. After you have ready the toast and the mushrooms, layer your ingredients.
3. Spread two tablespoons of hummus on each slice of toast, then add some blistered tomatoes, followed by bacon bits of vegan mushroom, cracked pepper, herbs and sea salt.
4. For every piece of toast, repeat the process.

16) Strawberry and Banana Muffins

Yield: 12 muffins

Ingredients:
- Non-dairy milk: ¾ cup
- Apple cider vinegar: 1 teaspoon
- Oat flour: 2 cups
- Sweet white rice flour: 1/3 cup
- Cornstarch powder: 1 tablespoon
- Baking powder: 3 teaspoons
- Salt: ½ teaspoon
- Ripe bananas: 2, mashed
- Maple syrup: 1/3 cup
- Melted coconut oil: 2 tablespoons
- Flax-meal: 1 tablespoon
- Vanilla extract: 1 teaspoon
- Chopped strawberries: 1 cup
- Vegan brown sugar or Coconut sugar: 1/3 cup

Instructions:
1. Set the oven to 350 ° F (175 ° C) and preheat it. Use paper liners to line a 12-cup muffin tray.
2. Combine the apple cider vinegar with a cup of milk and set aside.
3. Mix the oat flour, cornstarch, white rice flour, baking powder and salt and whisk together in a large bowl until thoroughly mixed.
4. In a medium bowl blend the maple syrup, bananas, coconut oil, vanilla extract and flax meal with the milk mixture. Put the wet ingredients and dry ingredients together in a bowl and stir until well combined. Fold in the coconut sugar and strawberries.
5. Pour the batter into the 12 muffins tray. Bake for 20 minutes, just until the top is firm and golden. Remove the tray from the oven. Rest aside the muffins to cool down before serving. Leftovers can be stored for 3 to 4 days, refrigerated or at room temperature.

17) Burritos filled with Tofu

Breakfast burritos loaded with scrambled tofu, onions, spinach and avocados make a perfect vegan breakfast rich in protein.

Prep Time: 5-6 minutes | Cook Time: 20 minutes | Total Time: 25 minutes| Calories: 500 kcal

Ingredients:
- Coconut oil or extra virgin olive: 1 tablespoon
- Potatoes: 3/4 cup, 1/2-inch diced
- Extra-firm organic tofu: 5 oz, about 3/4 cup, drained, and crumbled.
- Ground turmeric: 1/4 teaspoon
- Garlic powder: 1/4 teaspoon
- Sea salt: 1/4 teaspoon
- Nutritional yeast: 1 tablespoon
- Unsweetened non-dairy milk: 2 tablespoons
- Tortilla: 1 large, warmed
- Avocado: 1/4 peeled and sliced
- Baby spinach: /3 cup, fresh
- Salsa of your choice

Instructions:
1. Add a quarter of the oil in a saucepan, and place it over medium heat, to roast the potatoes. Add in the potatoes seasoned with salt and pepper. Cook for about 5 minutes, until crispy and golden brown.
2. Add 1 cup of water in a pan and cover it, about 10 minutes, to steam the potatoes the rest of the way. If the potatoes are not yet moist and the water has evaporated, add more water. Put the potatoes into a pan.
3. In the same pan heat, the oil remained over medium heat, to make the tofu scramble. Add drained and crumbled tofu, garlic, turmeric, nutritional yeast and salt.
4. Cook for 3 minutes, with frequent stirring. Add the milk and cook for another minute, to make the scramble fluffy.
5. Season with salt and pepper.
6. Put the potatoes, tofu scramble, greens and avocado over the tortilla to assemble the burrito. Roll up a side of the tortilla as tightly as you can over the fillings. Tuck over the short ends, and tie up. For a quick crunch, you can grill the outside of the burrito, or eat it right away. Use salsa for serving.

18) Sweet Potato Millet Pancakes

Prep Time: 10-12 mins| Cook Time: 20 mins| Total Time: 30 mins

Ingredients:
- Millet flour: 1/2 cup
- All-purpose flour: 1 cup, gluten-free or spelt
- Baking powder: 2 teaspoons
- Salt: 1/4 teaspoon
- Ground cinnamon: 1 teaspoon
- Ground nutmeg: 1/4 teaspoon
- Cane sugar: 2 tablespoons

- Apple cider vinegar: 1 teaspoon
- Almond milk: 1 1/4 - 1 1/2 cups start by using 1 1/4 cups
- Vegetable oil: 1 tablespoon
- Sweet potato puree: 3/4 cup

Instructions:
1. Oil a broad skillet or griddle lightly.
2. Whisk the flours, baking powder, nutmeg, salt, cinnamon, and sugar together in a bowl.
3. Mix the apple cider vinegar with 1 1/4 tablespoon almond milk.
4. Add vegetable oil and potato puree.
5. Blend the wet and dry ingredients, until thoroughly combined.
6. If the batter is too thick, add more almond milk, 2 tbsps at a time, until pancakes have the correct consistency.
7. Rest aside the batter and in the meanwhile heat the skillet over medium heat.
8. In 1/4-cup scoops, when the skillet is hot, add the batter.
9. Cook the pancakes until tiny bubbles show up on the surface of each pancake, and the bottom is firm.
10. Turn the pancakes, and let them cook for another 2 minutes on the other side, or until pancakes are golden and fluffy on both sides. Switch the pancakes to a rack or plate for cooling. Repeat the process with remaining mixture.

19) Tater Tot Waffles

Yes, you can use a waffle iron to turn tater tots into the perfect waffles ever! Breakfast is not getting any easier or better.

Yield: 8 Servings| Prep time: 10 minutes| Cook time: 20 minutes| Total time: 30 minutes

Ingredients:
- Frozen and thawed tater tots: 1 (32-ounce) bag
- Cajun seasoning: 1 tablespoon fine
- Salt or freshly ground black pepper to taste.
- Parsley leaves: 2 tablespoons, fresh and chopped

Instructions:
1. Preheat waffle iron to medium heat. Lightly oil the waffle iron's top and bottom, or brush with non-stick spray.
2. Working in lots, pouring tater tots into the waffle iron in one even layer. Sprinkle Cajun seasoning and salt and pepper.
3. Cover, press down firmly to flatten, and cook until crisp and golden brown, around 5-6 minutes or until you achieve desired crispness.
4. Repeat the process with remaining tater tots, spraying as needed more non-stick spray.
5. Serve with parsley.

20) Black Bean and Sweet Potato Burritos

Prep Time: 5-6 mins| Cook Time: 20 mins |Yield: 5 burritos

Ingredients:

- Yellow Onion: 1, diced
- Sweet Potatoes: 3, medium to large, peeled and diced.
- Black Beans: 1 cup
- Salsa of choice: 1 cup
- Fresh Spinach: 2 cups
- Wraps of your choice

Instructions:
1. Wash, peel and cut all vegetables.
2. In a large saucepan add 1/2 cup of water and add sweet potatoes and diced onions. Cook for 5-7 minutes over medium to high heat.
3. Reduce the heat to low and add salsa and black beans. If required, add few drops of water too. Cook for another 10 to 15 minutes or until the potatoes are moist and tender. Turn the heat off and let the bean mixture and sweet potatoes to cool.
4. Make the burritos using any wraps. Spoon the mixture into the wraps and tuck the sides. If you like you can add spinach as well.
5. Serve warm.

2.2. Vegan Soups, Salads and Snacks Recipes
Snacks:
Such portable, protein-rich, fiber-rich, vegan snacks are easy choices for helping to alleviate meal hunger.

1) Cocoa Strawberry balls
Calories: 362 kcal
Ingredients:
- Frozen strawberries: 2 x 15g packets
- Berry muesli: 1 1/2 cups, toasted
- Almond butter: 1/3 cup
- Strawberry jam: 2 tablespoons
- Cocoa powder: 1 tablespoon, dutch-processed

Instructions:
1. Put aside 6 frozen-dried strawberries. Chop the rest of the strawberries, roughly. Blend muesli in a hand blender until finely chopped.
2. Add the jam, almond butter, cocoa, and the chopped strawberries in a blender and blend until well combined. Make small balls of the blended mixture.
3. Crush in a bowl, strawberries that were reserved. Roll the balls you made in the crushed strawberries to coat all over.
4. Place the balls onto a plate. Serve.

2) Guacamole with Crackers
Cook Time: 5-10 minutes| Serves: 1 person
Ingredients:
- Ripe avocados: 2 mediums, peeled and chopped
- Red onion: 1/3 cup, chopped

- Fresh cilantro: 1/4 cup chopped
- Lime juice: 2 tablespoons
- Jalapeño pepper: 1/2 fresh, finely chopped
- Salt: 1/4 teaspoon
- Pepper: 1/8 teaspoon
- Garlic: 1 clove, minced
- Plum tomato: 1/2 cup, chopped

Instructions:
1. Take a bowl and mash the avocados in it using a fork. Add cilantro, onion, lime juice, salt, jalapeno pepper and garlic. Mix well.
2. Add 1/2 cup tomato. Use more tomatoes to garnish, if desired. Serve with crackers.

3) Edamame with Sea Salt

This Salted Edamame is inspired by a famous Japanese restaurant and takes 15 minutes and 2 simple ingredients to prepare. Enjoy as a midday snack!

Ingredients:
- Fresh or frozen soybeans
- Sea Salt to Taste

Instructions:
1. Bring a half-filled medium-sized saucepan of water to boil.
2. Add soybeans, and cook for five minutes.
3. Drain soybeans and sprinkle the salt on top. Enjoy!!

4) Roasted Chickpeas

Yield: 2 cups| Calories: 179

Ingredients:
- Chickpeas: 2 cans (15-ounce)
- Olive oil: 2 tablespoons
- Kosher salt: 1 teaspoon
- Spices or fresh herbs: 2 to 4 teaspoons (chilli powder, garam masala, curry powder, smoked paprika, cumin, thyme, rosemary, or other favorite herbs and spices)

Instructions:
1. Set the oven to 400 ° F and preheat it.
2. Wash the chickpeas, drain and pat dry.
3. Spray some olive oil over the chickpeas and sprinkle some salt.
4. Arrange the chickpeas on a rack and put it in the oven for 20-30 minutes.
5. Remove the chickpeas from the oven when golden and crispy from outside, and soft in the inside.
6. Sprinkle the spices over the chickpeas and serve.

5) Strawberry Rolls

Prep Time: 15 minutes| Cook Time: 4 hours| Total time: 4.5 hours| Yield: 10 rolls| Calories: 24kcal per roll

Ingredients:
- Strawberries: 4 cups
- Lemon Juice: 1 tablespoon
- Maple syrup: 1 tablespoon

Instructions:
1. Set the oven to 170° F and preheat it. Line a parchment paper on a baking pan.
2. Blend the strawberries, the maple syrup and lemon juice until smooth in a high-speed blender.
3. Spread the mixture over the baking pan and uniformly scatter to cover the whole baking sheet.
4. Bake for 5-6 hours, rotating halfway through the oven.
5. Remove from the oven when they are not soft or sticky anymore. Put them in the refrigerator to chill. Once chilled, cut in blocks, make rolls and serve.

6) Hummus and Veggies

The next time your kids ask for a snack, do not hand them the chips and dips. Instead, serve them some creamy and healthy hummus. Made of chickpeas, it is healthier than cream-filled dips. Plus, much better in taste!

Calories: 71.1 kcal

Ingredients:
- Fresh veggies of your choice
- Store-bought hummus

Instructions:
1. Wash and dry the vegetables.
2. Dice them into pieces of bite-size. Some vegetables, such as baby carrots and snap peas, need not be sliced.
3. Place 2 tbsps. of hummus on the plate of each person. Dip bits of your favorite veggies into hummus, and enjoy!

7) Rice Cakes and Avocado

These rice cakes are topped with spicy tomato jam and sliced avocados. A sprinkle of pepper and salt finishes off this easy yet fulfilling snack.

Instructions:
- Avocado: ½ small avocado, thinly sliced
- Rice cakes: 2
- Spicy Tomato Jam: ¼ cup
- Freshly ground black pepper (optional)
- Sea Salt (optional)

Directions:
1. Mash the avocados and spoon it on each rice cake.
2. Top with spicy tomato jam and sprinkle some pepper and salt as desired. Serve immediately!

8) Popcorn with Nutritional Yeast

The perfect Nooch popcorns are made without any artificial ingredient and are organic, gluten-free, and dairy-free.

Prep Time: 1 minute| Cook Time: 4 minutes| Total Time: 5 minutes| Yield: 8 cups of popcorns.

Ingredients:
- Nutritional yeast: 1/3 cup
- Fine sea salt: 1 teaspoon or more/less to taste
- Coconut oil: 3 tablespoons
- Popcorn kernels: 1/2 cup

Instructions:
1. Add salt and the nutritional yeast in a container and cover the lid. Rest aside.
2. Heat up the oil over moderate heat in a saucepan and put 4-5 kernels in it.
3. When the kernels start popping up, add the rest of the kernels in a single layer in the pan.
4. Cover the lid, and shake it, so the kernels get covered with the oil.
5. Shake the pan after every 15-20 seconds.
6. When the popping of kernels slows down and a few seconds left between pops, transfer the popcorns to the container immediately.
7. Cover with a lid, and shake it for 10-15 seconds, so the popcorns get coated in the dressing.
8. Serve and enjoy!

9) Nutty Fruit Bars

These nutty fruit bars are a tastier alternative to granola bars. Use of the Medjool dates in the recipe is a must; otherwise, the bars will be dry.

Total Time: 50 Mins| Yield: 16 Bars| Calories: 149 kcal

Ingredients:
- Chopped almonds: 1/3 cup
- Chopped pecans: 1/3 cup
- Honey: 1/2 cup
- Medjool dates: 3/4 cup, pitted
- Cinnamon: 1 teaspoon
- Regular rolled oats: 2 1/2 cups
- Dried cranberries: 1/2 cup
- Chopped dried apples: 1/2 cup

Directions:
1. Set the oven to 325 ° C and preheat it. Line a parchment paper on a baking tray and spread nuts on it. Bake for 10-12 minutes, until slightly golden.
2. Microwave honey until it turns into a thin syrup-like consistency. Blend cinnamon, honey, oats, and dates in a blender until the oats are roughly chopped.
3. Scrape the mixture of oat into a small bowl. Add cranberries, nuts and apples.

4. Shape the mixture into small balls. Spread the foil on a tray and spray some oil on the foil. Using damp hands, gently pat the balls onto the foil into small rectangles.
5. Freeze, for about 20-25 minutes, until the rectangles are firm enough to serve.
6. If you like them to be moist then let the bars in the refrigerator for a day.

10) Salsa with Tortilla Chips

Total Time: 20 minutes| Prep Time: 20-22 minutes| Yield: about 2 cups

Ingredients:
- Tomatoes: 4 ripe or plum, cored and roughly chopped
- Onion: 1/2 medium-sized (about 3 tablespoons), finely chopped
- Jalapeno: 1, minced
- Fresh coriander: 1/4 cup, chopped
- Kosher salt to taste
- Freshly ground black pepper
- Tortilla Chips

Directions:
1. Mix the onion, tomatoes, jalapeno, and coriander, in a small bowl. Sprinkle some salt and pepper. Use plastic wrap to cover and rest aside for almost an hour. Serve with tortilla chips.

Soups:

The simple chili soup recipe topped the list when it comes to simple and tasty vegan soup recipes. Zucchini soup, cabbage lentil soup, spring vegetable soup and potato soup are some of the other favorites that you can enjoy as dinner or snacks.

1) Cabbage Lentil Soup

A delicious soup made with two healthy ingredients cabbage and lentils, and carefully picked nutritious herbs and spices, all come together in just 20 minutes in one bowl!

Prep Time: 15 mins| Cook Time: 60 mins| Total Time: 1 hour 15 mins| Yield: 4

Ingredients:
- Coconut oil: 1/2 tablespoon
- Chopped onion: 1 cup
- Minced garlic: 1/2 tablespoon
- Apple cider vinegar: 1 tablespoon + 1/2 tablespoon extra (optional)
- Basil: 1 teaspoon
- Bay leaf: 1
- Vegetable stock (low sodium): 4 cups
- Miso: 1 teaspoon
- Tomatoes: 1 28 oz canned, peeled and crushed with your hands
- Green cabbage: 1/2 head
- Sriracha: 1/2 teaspoon
- Green lentils: 1 1/3 cup, cooked
- Sea salt, and ground pepper

Instructions:

1. Heat the coconut oil in a broad skillet over medium heat.
2. Add onions, stir and cook until the onion is tender.
3. Add garlic, basil and bay leaf; cook for 2 minutes.
4. To deglaze the pot, apply 1 tablespoon of apple cider vinegar.
5. Add stock, cabbage, canned tomatoes, sriracha and miso.
6. Bring the stock to boil. Reduce flame, and simmer for a total of 30 minutes.
7. Add lentils and simmer for another 20 minutes.
8. For seasoning use salt, pepper and apple cider vinegar.

2) Butternut Squash Soup

It is insanely easy to prepare and so incredibly cozy and tasty, naturally gluten-free and vegan.

Prep time: 20-22 minutes| Cook time: 30 minutes| Total time: 50-52 minutes| yield: 6 -8 Servings

Ingredients:
- Vegetable stock: 2 cups
- Garlic: 4 cloves, peeled and minced
- Carrot: 1, roughly chopped
- Granny Smith apple: 1, cored and chopped
- Butternut squash: 1 medium, and diced
- White onion: 1, roughly chopped
- 1 sprig fresh sage
- Salt: 1/2 teaspoon
- Ground black pepper: 1/4 teaspoon
- Cayenne: 1/8 teaspoon
- Nutmeg and ground cinnamon: a pinch
- Unsweetened coconut milk: 1/2 cup canned
- Garnishes (optional): smoked paprika Or extra coconut milk

Instructions:
1. In a small (4-quarters) slow cooker or big (6-quarters) slow cooker add vegetable stock, garlic, apple, butternut squash, carrot, salt, pepper, sage, cayenne, onion, nutmeg and cinnamon. Toss well.
2. Cook at medium heat for 6-7 hours or at high heat for 3-4 hours, just until the squash is fully tender and easily mashed with a fork.
3. Remove the sage, and discard it. Add the coconut milk.
4. Puree the soup until smooth, with an electric mixer.
5. Add cayenne and salt and pepper to taste, and season as needed.
6. Serve dry, top with the garnishes you want.

3) Vegan Roasted Red Pepper and Ginger Soup

It is a balanced and tasty carrot and red pepper soup that is made in the instant pot. This gluten-free, vegan soup has strong, bold flavors from the roasting of carrots and red peppers.

Prep Time: 5-6 minutes| Cook Time: 55 minutes| Total Time: 1 hour| Servings: 3| Calories: 171kcal

Ingredients:
- Carrots: 4
- Red pepper: 2, remove stem and seeds, diced into large pieces
- Onion: 1/2, cut into large pieces
- Garlic: 4 cloves
- Olive oil: 2 tablespoons, divided
- Vegetable Broth: 3 cups
- Salt: 1 teaspoon, divided
- 1 Bay leaf
- Ground cumin: 1 teaspoon
- Garnishing:
- Black pepper: 1/4 teaspoon (optional)
- Cilantro to garnish: 3 tablespoons (optional)
- Sesame seeds: 1/2 teaspoon (optional)

Instructions:

To roast veggies:
1. Set the oven temperature to 400° F. Place red peppers and carrots (cut side down) in a layer onto a foiled baking tray.
2. Spray some olive oil and sprinkle a little salt over the tray.
3. Cook in the oven for 30 minutes. Remove from the frying pan. Rest aside the peppers to cool so that that blackened skin can be peeled easily.
4. Preparing the soup:
5. Set the instant pot in sauté mode, press start and let it heat up.
6. Stir in olive oil, garlic, bay leaf and onions. Let them take around 3 minutes to sauté.
7. Add the broth, red peppers and the roasted carrots. Add salt and ground cumin. Close the lid.
8. On manual mode, start the instant pot for 3 minutes. Once the instant pot buzz, let the pressure release naturally.
9. Remove bay leaf. Blend the broth to a smooth consistency, using an immersion blender. Garnish with black pepper.
10. Garnish with sesame seeds and cilantro.

4) Kale and Tortellini Soup

A simple and flavorful tortellini cheese soup packed with kale, kidney beans and red bell pepper.

Prep Time: 10-12 minutes| Cook Time: 35 minutes| Total Time: 45- 47 minutes| Yield: 5 to 6 servings

Ingredients:
- Olive oil: 1 1/2 tablespoons
- Onion: 1 medium, chopped

- Red bell pepper: 1 medium, chopped
- Garlic: 2 cloves, minced
- Fire-roasted tomatoes: 1 (14-ounce) can, diced
- Red kidney beans: 1 can (15-ounce), drained and rinsed
- Vegetable broth (low sodium): 5 cups
- Red pepper flakes: 1/2 teaspoon
- Lemon juice: 1 tablespoon
- Salt: 1 teaspoon
- Dried basil: 1/2 teaspoon
- Dried parsley: 1/2 teaspoon
- Fresh cheese tortellini: 1 (about 10-ounce) package
- Lacinato kale: 1 (about 9-ounce) bunch, remove stems and crush leaves into pieces of bite-sized
- For serving: Parmesan or shredded mozzarella (optional)

Instructions:
1. Add the olive oil into a large stockpot and put over medium heat.
2. Add in pepper and onion when hot, and cook for around 5 to 7 minutes, until moist and tender.
3. Stir in the finely chopped garlic and cook until fragrant, for 30 seconds.
4. Put kidney beans, broth, salt, lemon juice, basil, red pepper flakes, and parsley into the diced tomatoes.
5. Stir and boil, then turn the heat low and allow for 15 minutes simmering.
6. Add the kale and the tortellini and proceed to cook for around 6 to 8 minutes or until tender.
7. Turn off the heat. As required, season with extra red pepper flakes and salt. Garnish with cheese.

5) Tomato and Rice Soup with Chickpeas

Serves: 2 to 3| Active Time: 25-27 minutes| Total Time: 40 minutes

Ingredients:
- Extra-virgin olive oil: 5 teaspoons
- Yellow onion: 1 small, diced
- Rainbow chard: 1 bunch, remove stems and chop into 1/2-inch pieces
- Garlic: 2 medium cloves, minced
- Tomatoes (can-crushed): 1 (28 ounces)
- Kosher salt
- Vegetable stock: 2 cups, low-sodium
- Canned chickpeas: 1 (15.5 ounces), drained and rinsed
- Basmati rice: 1/2 cup, cooked according to directions on the package
- Freshly ground black pepper

Directions:
1. Heat 2-3 teaspoons of oil over medium heat in a small saucepan.

2. Add chard stems (not leaves) and onions and sauté for around 5 minutes, until the onions are translucent and the stems are soft.
3. Adding the minced garlic, cook for another 1 minute, stirring until fragrant. Sprinkle with salt and add tomatoes.
4. Cook for 2-3 minutes, then stir in stock. Bring stock to boil, reduce to a simmer and cook for about 10 minutes, until slightly reduced.
5. Heat remaining two tsp of oil over high heat in a large saucepan pan until the oil is shimmering and hot.
6. Add chickpeas, sprinkle with salt and cook over medium-high heat for around 3 minutes, until crispy and browned.
7. Use a paper towel to drain, then stir in rice and soup.
8. Add chard leaves in batches over medium-high heat in soup, wait for the leaves to be soft and wilted before adding more.
9. Simmer for 1 minute to cook everywhere through, then serve with salt and pepper seasoning.

6) Vegan Zucchini Soup

Prep Time: 5-6 minutes| Cook Time: 15 minutes| Total Time: 20 minutes| Servings: 4 bowls| Calories: 251kcal| Calories: 251kcal

Ingredients:
- Raw cashews: 1 cup
- Vegetable stock: 3 ½ cups
- Peeled zucchini: 1 kilogram, roughly chopped
- Sea salt (optional)
- Pepper (optional)
- Vegan butter spread: 1 tablespoon (optional)

Instructions:
1. Put the stock, cashews and peeled zucchini over low-medium heat into a casserole, and bring to boil.
2. Cook for 12-15 minutes until the zucchini and cashews are tender.
3. Turn off the heat and add the soup into a blender. Add the vegan butter and sprinkle salt and pepper. Blend until the soup is creamy and thick.

7) Potato Soup

Prep Time: 5-6 minutes| Cook Time: 20 minutes| Total Time: 25 minutes| Makes: 2 servings| Calories: 255kcal

Ingredients:
- Potatoes: 450 g, cut into bite-sized chunks
- Onions: 2 larges, roughly chopped
- Vegetable broth: 4 cups
- Black pepper: a few grinds (optional)

Instructions:
1. Pour the vegetable stock in a deep saucepan and bring to a simmer.
2. Add onion and potato, cover, and cook for 20-25 minutes.

3. Set it aside to cool after turning the heat off. Once cool transfer the soup to blender and blend until smooth.
4. For serving, use black pepper grinds.

8) Spring Vegetables Soup

Prep Time: 10-12 minutes| Cook Time: 30-35 minutes| Total Time: 40 minutes| Servings: 5 Portions Calories: 152 kcal

Ingredients:
- Carrots: 3
- Celery Stalks: 3
- Potatoes: 2, large
- Frozen/Fresh Peas: 1 cup
- Onion: 1, small
- Salt to taste
- Vegetable Stock Cube: 1
- Sunflower Oil: 2 tablespoons

Instructions
1. Slice the onion after peeling it. Sauté the onion in a pan for 3-4 minutes over medium heat, stirring frequently.
2. Cut slices of celery, carrots and potatoes after peeling them. Sauté them for about 2-3 minutes in the pan along with the peas. Add 1.5 litres of water. Add 2 teaspoons of salt and bring the soup to boil.
3. Stir in the cube of vegetable stock and lower the heat.
4. Cook the soup for 30-35 minutes, then transfer to dishes and serve warm.

9) Pumpkin Soup

Serves: 4

Ingredients:
- Butternut pumpkin: 1 small, peeled, deseeded & diced, (weighs about 2.6 kg/ 6 pounds)
- Hot water: 900ml
- Thai Green Curry Paste: 1 tablespoon
- Coconut milk: 135ml

Instructions:
1. Add chopped pumpkin in a saucepan. Then add around 1 litre of boiling water, enough to cover the pumpkin.
2. Cover the lid and cook the pumpkin, until it is mash-able.
3. Set it aside after turning off the heat. Once cool blend the pumpkin until a smooth and creamy consistency is achieved.
4. Transfer the soup back in the saucepan and boil the soup over low-medium heat. Add coconut milk and green curry paste and mix. Continue to cook until the desired consistency of the soup is achieved. Sprinkle salt and pepper. Garnish with chili flakes and chopped coriander.

10) Easy Chili Soup

Prep Time: 5-10 minutes| Cook Time: 30-35 Minutes| Total Time: 35 Minutes| Serves: 6|

Ingredients:
- Ground beef: 1 pound, cooked and drained
- Chilli beans: Can of 15 ounces, undrained
- Tomatoes with green chilies: 10 ounce can, diced
- Toppings:
- Sour Cream
- Cilantro
- Tortilla Chips
- Green Onions

Instructions:
1. Combine the beans, meat and tomatoes in a water-filled pot. Bring to a boil over low-moderate heat, then lower the heat and simmer for about 30 minutes.
2. Season with salt and pepper. Top with sour cream and cheese.

Salads:

Below is a list of the yummy vegan salad recipes that include a wide variety of legumes, vegetables, and grains to make a delicious and mouthwatering addition to every vegan diet.

1) Quinoa and Smoked Tofu Salad

This salad is loaded with heart-healthy and power ingredients — whole grains legumes, soy-based tofu, quinoa, and plenty of healthy veggies.

Total Time: 35 mins| Servings: 6 | Calorie: 244kcal

Ingredients:
- Water: 2 cups
- Salt: ¾ teaspoon, divided
- Quinoa: 1 cup, rinsed well
- Lemon juice: ¼ cup
- Extra-virgin olive oil: 3 tablespoons
- Garlic: 2 small cloves, minced
- Freshly ground pepper: ¼ teaspoon
- Baked smoked tofu: 1 6- or 8-ounce package, diced
- Yellow bell pepper: 1 small, diced
- Grape tomatoes: 1 cup, halved
- Cucumber: 1 cup, diced
- Fresh parsley: ½ cup, chopped
- Fresh mint: ½ cup, chopped

Directions:
1. In a saucepan, add water and ½ teaspoon salt and bring it to boil. Add the quinoa and boil again for 15 to 18 minutes until the water is evaporated.
2. Spread the quinoa over a foiled baking sheet and rest aside for 10 minutes to cool.
3. In a wide cup, whisk together lemon juice, butter, garlic, the remaining 1/4 tsp salt and pepper.

4. Add the tofu, cooled quinoa, bell pepper, cucumber, tomatoes, parsley, and mint; mix well and serve.

2) Roasted Veggie Mason Jar Salad

Active Time: 5 minutes| Total Time: 5-6 minutes| Servings: 1 Per Serving: 400 calories;

This mason jar vegan salad is easy to prepare for lunch and snack as well. Layer the creamy cashew sauce at the bottom of the jar so that the time you are ready to eat, your power salad will not get wilted.

Ingredients:
- Vegan Cashew Sauce: 2 tablespoons
- Roasted tofu: 1 cup (see associated recipes)
- Pumpkin seeds: 1 tablespoon
- Roasted vegetables: 1 cup
- Mixed greens: 2 cups

Directions:
1. Follow the order to layer the ingredients into a 4-cup jar: sauce, pumpkin seeds, tofu, greens and vegetables. Close firmly, and toss the jar slightly.

3) Kale, Carrot & Apple Salad

Green Lacinato kale is the highlight of this balanced kale salad, tossed with mustard, maple syrup and apple cider vinaigrette and stuffed with crunchy apples.

Total: 30 mins| Servings: 12| Calories: 75kcal

Ingredients:

For the Dressing:
- For Cider Vinaigrette:
- Shallot: 1 small, chopped
- Cider vinegar: ¼ cup
- Extra-virgin olive oil: 3 tablespoons
- Apple cider: 2 tablespoons
- Whole-grain mustard: 1 ½ tablespoon
- Pure maple syrup: 2 teaspoons
- Salt: ½ teaspoon
- Ground pepper to taste

For Salad:
- Lacinato kale: 1-2 large bunches, 10 cups coarsely chopped
- 2 sweet-tart apples, cut into matchsticks
- Carrots: 3 cups, cut in the shape of a matchstick
- Radishes: 1 cup, cut like matchsticks
- Parsley leaves: ¾ cup, coarsely chopped

Directions:
1. To make the vinaigrette: Take a blender and blend shallot, sugar, vinegar, cinnamon, maple syrup, salt and pepper and mustard, until creamy and smooth.

2. To make the salad: Take a large bowl, mix kale, carrots, apples, radishes, and parsley. Put the dressing over the salad, cover the lid of the bowl, shake it and then serve it.

Tips:
3. Marinate the dressing on kale for about 30 minutes before serving.
4. The strong kale leaves will not wilt out of the dressing and will taste much better after being marinated in it.

4) White Bean and Veggie Salad

This salad combines creamy avocado and white beans to satisfy your taste buds. You can mix it with various seasonal veggies as well.

Active: 10 minutes| Total: 10-12 minutes| Servings: 1| Calories: 360kcal

Ingredients:
- Mixed salad greens: 2 cups
- Veggies you like: ¾ cup
- Canned white beans: ⅓ cup, rinsed and drained
- Avocado: ½, diced
- Red-wine vinegar: 1 tablespoon
- Extra-virgin olive oil: 2 teaspoons
- Kosher salt: ¼ teaspoon
- Freshly ground pepper to taste

Directions:
1. Take a medium-sized bowl, and mix vegetables, tomatoes, avocado, and beans in it. Drizzle some oil and vinegar, and use salt and pepper as seasoning. Toss the salad, so it is well combined. Serve!

5) Quinoa Chickpea Salad with Roasted Red Pepper Hummus Dressing

This nutritious vegan salad is packed with the power of plant-based ingredients: Quinoa, chickpeas and hummus.

Active: 10 minutes| Total: 10-12 minutes| Servings: 1| Calories: 379 c

Ingredients:
- Hummus: 2 tablespoons, original OR roasted red pepper flavor
- Lemon juice: 2 tablespoons
- Roasted red pepper: 1 tablespoon chopped
- Mixed salad greens: 2 cups
- Cooked quinoa: ½ cup
- Chickpeas, rinsed: ½ cup
- Unsalted sunflower seeds: 1 tablespoon
- Chopped fresh parsley: 1 tablespoon
- Pinch of salt
- Pinch of ground pepper

Directions:
1. In a medium bowl mix together the hummus, red peppers and lemon juice. Add water into the dressing to thin it to desired consistency.

2. Take a large bowl and add beans, chickpeas, and quinoa in it. Top with parsley, sunflower seeds, and salt and pepper. Pour the dressing on it and serve.

6) Mexican salad with tortilla croutons

Prep Time: 10-12 minutes| Cook Time: 12 minutes| Serves: 4| Calories: 337 kcal

Ingredients:
- Flour tortillas: 3, cut into crouton-sized pieces
- Olive oil: 1 tablespoon
- Cajun seasoning: 1 teaspoon
- Iceberg lettuce: 1, shredded
- Black bean: Can of 400g, rinsed and drained
- Pack cherry tomato: 200g, halved
- Avocados: 2, peeled and sliced
- Juice of 1 lime
- Coriander leaves: ½ bunch

Instructions:
1. Preheat oven to 200C/180C.
2. Put the pieces of tortillas on a baking tray, toss with the oil and sprinkle the seasoning, then cook until crispy for 10 minutes.
3. Add the beans, iceberg, tomatoes, and avocados tossed in lime juice into a bowl.
4. Toss the salad in the dressing. Serve with the cilantro and croutons.

7) Spinach and Apple Salad

Prep Time: 10 minutes| Serves: 4 persons

Ingredients:
- Glazed Walnuts: 1/2 cup
- Balsamic Dressing
- Apple: 1
- Ripe pear: 1
- Baby spinach leaves: 3 cups
- Mixed greens: 3 cups

Instructions:
1. Keep Walnuts or Pecans Glazed.
2. Meanwhile, prepare the salad.
3. Cut thin slices of pear and apples.
4. Place the veggies on serving dish and add pears, apples and walnuts on top. Serve after pouring the store-bought balsamic dressing over the salad.

8) Hummus Salad Dressing

Prep Time: 5 Minutes| Yield: 1-2 servings

Ingredients:
- Garlic Hummus: ½ cup
- Dijon Mustard: 1 tablespoon
- Juice of ½ Lemon
- Filtered Water: 2–4 tablespoons

Instructions:
1. Add the mustard, hummus and Lemon Juice to a bowl and mix with a spoon.
2. Add 1 tablespoon of water until the desired consistency is achieved, then serve with your favorite salad.

9) Mediterranean Salad

Prep Time: 10-12 minutes| Total Time: 15 minutes| Yield: serves 4 to 6 people

Ingredients:
- Roma tomatoes: 6 (about 3 cups), diced
- Cucumber: 1 large, diced
- Fresh parsley leaves: 15-20 g, chopped
- salt, to taste
- Black pepper: 1/2 teaspoon
- Ground Sumac: 1 teaspoon
- Extra virgin olive oil: 2 tablespoons
- Lemon juice: 2 teaspoons

Instructions:
1. Layer a big salad bowl with the cucumbers, diced tomatoes and parsley. Add salt, and rest aside for about four minutes.
2. Add the other ingredients in the bowl and give it a quick toss. Allow the aromas to blend for a 4-5 minutes before serving.

10) Avocado Salad

Prep Time: 10 minutes

Ingredients:
- Cherry tomatoes: 1 cup, halved
- Avocados: 2, diced
- Marinated artichoke hearts: 1 jar (6.5 ounces), coarsely chopped

Instructions:
1. Add diced tomatoes and avocado in a mixing bowl.
2. Drain marinated artichoke hearts, and put aside the drained marinade.
3. Add chopped artichoke hearts in tomatoes and avocados and toss until well combined.
4. You can use the reserved marinade for flavor as desired.

2.3. Smoothies and Beverages

1) Simple Strawberry Smoothie

Ingredients:
- Frozen Strawberries: 1 cup
- Soymilk: 1 cup
- Soy yoghurt: 1/2 cup
- Orange Juice: 1 Cup

Instructions:
1. Blend all ingredients, gradually adding soymilk or orange juice to reach the desired thickness.

2) Carrot, Spinach and Ginger Juice

Ingredients:
- Carrots: 4
- Spinach: A handful
- Ginger: Thumb-sized chuck

Instructions:
1. First Juice carrots, then add ginger and blend, and finally add spinach to make a delicious juice!

3) Spinach, Mango and Banana Juice

Ingredients:
- Spinach: 2 cups, freshly washed
- Chilled water: 1/2 cup
- Mango: 1 large, peeled and sliced
- Banana, 1 large, frozen (peel & freeze the banana for 2 – 4 hours before blending)

Instructions:
1. Blend the water and spinach first until liquid & frothy, then add banana and mango, and blend well until smooth.

4) Grapefruit Mango Smoothie

Ingredients:
- Mango: 1 sliced and frozen
- Grapefruit: 1 cut into slices
- Grapefruit juice: 1/2 grapefruit or whole as you like

Instructions:
1. Blend all the ingredients, gradually adding water to reach the consistency you like.

5) Mango Carrot and Banana Basil Smoothie

Ingredients
- Mango: 1, peeled and sliced
- Carrots: 2, medium-sized
- Banana: 1 frozen
- Basil leaves: 4-6 leaves
- Soy Milk: 1 1/2 Cups
- Stevia: 1 (optional)
- Ice cubes: 3-4

Instructions:
1. Blend all the ingredients until smooth.

6) Carrot Cucumber Spinach Smoothie

Ingredients:
- Carrot juice: 3/4 cup
- Cucumber juice: 3/4 cup
- Spinach juice: 3/4 cup

- Silk Vanilla: 1/2 cup
- Ice to fill up the blender

Instructions:
2. Blend all the ingredients until smooth.

7) Gazpacho Delight

Ingredients:
- Tomato juice: 2 ½ cups
- Garlic: 2 cloves
- Onion: 2 tablespoons
- Cilantro: 2 teaspoons
- Red pepper flakes: 1 half teaspoon
- Spinach: 1 tablespoon
- Cumin: 1 teaspoon

Instructions:
1. Put all the ingredients in the blender and blend until smooth.

8) Green Lemonade

Ingredients:
- Celery: 2 stalks
- Kale: 1 bushel
- Apple: 1
- Cucumber: 1 2/3
- Lemonade: 1-3 cups

Instructions:
1. Put all the ingredients in the blender and blend until smooth.

9) Carrot Mango Spinach Smoothie

Ingredients:
- Banana: 1
- Spinach: A handful
- Coconut milk: 1/4 can
- Frozen mango: 1 cup
- Baby carrots: 3
- Cinnamon: A dash or two

Instructions:
2. Blend all the ingredients, gradually adding water to reach the consistency you like.

10) Mango Carrot Cooler

Ingredients:
- Mango: 1
- Carrot: 1
- Ice cubes

Instructions:
1. Boil carrots and chopped mangos in water until the two are well cooked.

2. Let it cool and blend with ice, cumin powder, a few mint leaves, lemon juice, sugar and a little salt. Pour in a glass and serve!

2.4. Lunch and Dinner Recipes

Vegan lunch and dinner meals can either be prepared upfront and frozen in the refrigerator for up to 4 or 5 days, or assembled ahead and prepared in a slow cooker, skillet or instant oven! Preparing for certain lunches and dinners is beneficial in minimizing the tension of mealtime and saving you money (less ordering or dining out!).

1) Tofu Tacos

Made with a bit of spicy tofu filling, these fast vegan tacos make a great weekend dinner. Load them with shredded cabbage, guacamole, and fresh fresh pico de gallo to keep them vegan.

Active Time: 30 minutes| Total: 30 minutes|Servings:4

Ingredients:
- 1 tablespoon chili powder
- Ground cumin: 1 teaspoon
- Dried oregano: ½ teaspoon
- Salt: ½ teaspoon
- Ground pepper: ¼ tablespoon
- Cinnamon ground $1/8$ teaspoon
- Extra-firm tofu: 1 block (14 to 16 ounces), cut into 1/2 "cubes
- Extra virgin olive oil: 3 Tablespoons of
- Chopped onion: ½ cup
- Garlic cloves, minced: 2 Big
- Black beans: 1 can (15 ounces)
- Cider Vinegar: 2 Teaspoons
- Chopped cilantro: ½ cup
- Corn tortillas: 8 warmed
- Shredded cabbage, guacamole and pico de gallo (optional)

Directions:
1. In a medium-sized bowl, mix cumin, chili powder, salt, oregano, cinnamon, and pepper. Add and toss tofu to coat the seasonings. Rest aside
2. Add 2 tbsps. of oil in a wide non-stick skillet and put it over medium-high heat. Add onion, stir and cook for about 3 minutes until it begins to soften. Add garlic, stir and cook for 1-2 minute.
3. Raise to medium-high heat and add tofu. Cook for around 10 minutes, stirring periodically, until browning begins.
4. Add beans, stir and cook for 3-4 minutes until heated through. Turn the heat off; Stir in cilantro and vinegar.
5. To serve, add tofu filling, about 1/3 cup to each tortilla. If needed, top with the cabbage, guacamole and pico de gallo.

2) Soya Beans Hummus Wraps

This simple hummus recipe is only enough for two wraps, but the hummus is so delicious that you may want to double it and tuck it away for snacking in your fridge.
Total Prep time: 30 mins | Servings: 2

Ingredients:
- Frozen soybeans shelled (generous 1 cup), thawed: 6 Ounces
- Lemon juice: 2 Tablespoons (divided)
- Extra virgin olive oil: 2 Tablespoons (divided)
- Tahini: 1 tablespoon
- Finely chopped clove garlic: 1 tiny
- Ground cumin: ¼ Tablespoon
- Salt: 1/4 tsp
- Ground pepper: ¼ teaspoon of
- Green cabbage: 1 Cup, thinly sliced
- Orange bell pepper: ¼ cup, thinly sliced
- Scallion, thin slices: 1/2
- Fresh chopped parsley: 2 Tablespoons
- Whole wheat tortilla: 2

Instructions:
1. In a food processor, mix beans, 1 tablespoon lemon juice, 1 tablespoon olive oil, tahini, garlic, cumin, 1/8 teaspoon pepper and salt. Pulse until smooth.
2. In a medium cup, whisk the remaining 1 tablespoon of lemon juice and oil with the remaining 1/8 teaspoon pepper. Add cabbage, pepper bell, scallion and parsley; stir to coat.
3. Place half of the bean hummus over each tortilla's lower third, and cover it with half of the cabbage mixture. Make a roll. Cut to serve in half, if needed.

3) Buddha Vegan Bowl

This basic bowl of grain has so many healthy ingredients: protein-packed chickpeas, sweet potatoes, creamy avocado and tahini dressing.
Active: 30 minutes| Total time: 30 minutes |Servings: 4

Ingredients:
- Sweet potato: 1 medium, cut into 1-inch pieces, peeled if desired.
- Olive oil: 3 tablespoons, divided
- Salt divided: ½ Teaspoon
- Ground pepper, (divided): 1/2 teaspoon
- Tahini: 2 tablespoons
- Water: 2 cups
- Lemon juice: 1 tablespoon
- Small, minced clove of garlic: 2 pieces
- Quinoa Cooked: 2 cups
- Chickpeas, rinsed, (15-ounce 1 can)
- Mature avocado, diced: 1
- New parsley or cilantro chopped: ¼ cup

Instructions:
1. Preheat oven to 425 F.
2. Toss the sweet potato in a small bowl with 1 spoonful of oil and 1/4 teaspoon of salt and pepper. Switch to a baking sheet with rims. Bake for 16 to 18 minutes, stirring once, until tender.
3. Meanwhile, whisk each salt and pepper in a small bowl with the remaining 2 tablespoons of oil, tahini, water, lemon juice, garlic and 1/4 teaspoon remaining.
4. Divide the quinoa into 4 bowls to serve. Fill with the sweet potato, chickpea and avocado in similar amounts. Drizzle with tahini. Sprinkle with cilantro (or parsley).

4) Tijuana Torta Sandwich

A torta in the Mexican style is much like a burrito, except that the "wrapper" is a hollow-out roll, instead of a tortilla. It is loaded here with mashed black spiced beans and quick guacamole. Bring this vegetarian version to a new level (and add calcium) by rubbing the Monterey Jack cheese onto the sandwich's bean side. Serve on the cob or Spanish rice with grilled corn.

Total time: 25 minutes| Servings: 4

Ingredients:
- Black beans, or rinsed pinto beans: 1 can 15-ounce
- Salsa: 3 Spoonful
- Pickled jalapeño: 1 tablespoon
- ½ teaspoon of cumin
- 1 Mature avocado, pitted
- Chopped onion: 2 tablespoons
- Lime juice: 1 tablespoon
- Whole grain Baguette: 1 16- to 20-inch long
- Shredded green cabbage: 1⅓ cups

Instructions:
1. In a small bowl, mix the salsa, mash beans, cumin and jalapeno. In another small bowl, mix onion, lime juice and avocado.
2. Dice the baguette into 5 equal pieces. Cut each piece horizontally in half. Take much of the soft bread out of the middle, and you are just left with the crust.
3. Divide bean paste, avocado mixture and cabbage equally between sandwiches. Cut through and serve in half.

5) Brown Rice Bowl with Roasted Vegetables

This basic recipe of brown rice, broccoli, onions and peppers with roasted butternut squash, cashew tahini creamy sauce, and tofu marinated in lime, is a safe and fulfilling vegan lunch.

Active time: 5 minutes | Total: 5 minutes | Servings: 1

Ingredients:
- Cooked brown rice: ½ cup
- Roasted vegetables: 1 Cup

- Roasted tofu: 1 Cup
- Scallions sliced: 2 Tablespoons
- Fresh cilantro chopped: 2 Tablespoons
- Creamy Vegan Cashew Sauce: 2 Tablespoons

Directions:
1) Put rice, beans, and tofu in a sealable bowl or 4-cup dish. Sprinkle with the cilantro and scallions. When ready to eat, top with a sauce made with cashew.

6) Nice Black Bean Chili and Sweet Potato

For two, this delicious vegetarian chili is pickled with black beans and sweet potatoes. Serve with some warm corn tortillas, and toss the salad with orange and avocado segments.

Total time: 30 Minutes | Servings: 2

Ingredients:
- Extra virgin olive oil: 1 tablespoon
- Finely diced onion: 1 medium size
- Sweet potato, chopped: 1 medium size
- Garlic, minced: 2 cloves
- Chili powder: 1 tablespoon
- Cumin ground: 2 teaspoons
- Ground Chipotle, Chile: 1/4 teaspoon
- Salt: $1/8$ teaspoon
- Water: 1⅓ cups
- Dry, rinsed black beans: 1 can (15-ounce)
- Diced tomatoes: 1 cup
- Lime juice: 2 teaspoons
- Fresh cilantro chopped: 2 tablespoons

Steps to prepare:
1. Using frying pan heat oil over moderate to low heat. Add onion and potato, and cook for 4-5 minutes, frequently stirring until the onion is slightly softened.
2. Add the garlic, cumin, chili powder, salt and chipotle and cook for about 30 seconds, continually stirring, until fragrant. Add water, bring to a boil, cover, rising heat to maintain a gentle boil and cook until the potato is moist and tender, for around 10 minutes.
3. Add beans, lime juice and tomatoes; raise heat to high, and return to simmer, often stirring. Reduce heat to hold a simmer and cook for around 4 minutes, until slightly reduced. Add cilantro and stir, and then remove from heat.

7) Thai Curry Noodles with Peanut

The Thai curry paste in this balanced peanut noodle recipe offers spicy kick-in-the-pants. If you have not yet tried kohlrabi, here is your excuse for buying it. The bulbous vegetable is related to the sprouts of broccoli and Brussels but has a milder, sweet taste and fabulous crunch.

Total time: 30 minutes | Servings: 4

Ingredients:

- Spaghetti of whole wheat: 8 Ounces
- Natural, smooth peanut butter: ½ cup
- Minced shallot: 1 small
- Curry paste Thai green, red, or yellow: 2 tablespoons
- Fresh ginger minced: 1 tablespoon
- Reduced-sodium soy sauce: 1 tablespoon
- Toasted sesame oil: 2 teaspoons
- Salt: ¼ teaspoon
- Frozen edamame: ½ cup, thawed
- Red peppered bell: 1 medium, cut into matchsticks
- Kohlrabi broccoli: 1 Cup, peeled, stems removed
- Fresh cilantro(optional): ¼ cup, peeled

Directions:
1. Fill a medium saucepan of water and bring it to boil. Remove spaghetti and cook according to the instructions on the box. Reserve the liquid for 1/4 cup, then drain the spaghetti and rinse well with cold water.
2. In a big cup, whisk the reserved spaghetti water, peanut butter, shallot, curry paste, ginger, soya sauce, oil and salt. Add the rice, edamame, pepper bell, and kohlrabi (or stem broccoli); mix well to coat. If desired, serve topped with cilantro.

8) Vegetarian Lettuce Wraps

Stuff crisp lettuce leaves inspired by PF Chang's popular lettuce wraps with a savory filling. This low-carb wraps made with tofu, mushrooms and radish daikon are a simple vegetarian dinner to carry out beats! For additional snap, garnish the wraps with julienned carrots.

Prep Time: 40 minutes | Full Time: 40 minutes | Servings: 4

Ingredients:
- Rice vinegar: 3 tablespoons
- Hoisin sauce: 2 tablespoons
- Low-sodium soy sauce: 2 tablespoons
- Sesame oil: 1 teaspoon
- Crushed red potatoes: ¼ teaspoon
- Extra-firm tofu: 1 (14 ounces)
- Canola oil: 1 tablespoon
- White mushrooms: 8 ounces, finely chopped
- Daikon radish: 1 cup finely chopped
- Garlic cloves, minced: 3 Big
- Grated ginger: 1 spoonful
- Scallions, sliced: 4
- Big Bibb or iceberg Lettuce leaves: 8 leaves
- (Optional) Julienned Carrots

Directions:

1. In a small bowl, combine vinegar, hoisin, soya sauce, sesame oil and crushed red pepper and set aside.
2. Slice the tofu horizontally in half. Remove as much water as possible, pressing the tofu slices between paper towels. Crumble it.
3. Heat the canola oil over medium to high heat in a large non-stick skillet. Add the crumbled tofu; cook, stir and break into smaller bits, about 5 minutes before you start browning.
1) Add mushrooms; continue cooking and stirring for about 3 minutes, until any liquid has evaporated.
2) Add ginger, garlic daikon and scallions. Add the reserved sauce; cook for about 2 minutes, stirring, until well mixed and heated through.
3) Spoon each lettuce leaf with a little 1/2 cup tofu mixture. When needed, top with carrots.

9) Purple Artichoke Pizza & Asparagus

Lemon and pecorino top off this tasty, easy home-made pizza which gets vibrant asparagus and artichoke color. Shiso is a mint family Fuzzy-leafed herb that is used in several Asian cuisines. It is rising in their gardens by devoted fans; look for it on Asian and farmer's markets.

Preparation Time: 24-25 Minutes |Servings: 5

Ingredients:
- Cornmeal: 1 tablespoon
- Whole-wheat pizza dough, at room temperature: 1 pound
- Extra-virgin olive oil, divided: 2 tablespoons
- Garlic sliced: 2 cloves
- kosher salt divided: ¼ teaspoon
- Crushed red pepper: ⅛ teaspoon
- Mozzarella cheese: 1½ cups shredded part-skim
- Baby purple artichokes: 2
- Lemon zest: 1 teaspoon
- Lemon juice: 2 tablespoons
- Purple asparagus: 8 ounces, trimmed
- Grated pecorino cheese: 2 ounces (1/2 cup)
- Ground pepper: ¼ teaspoon
- Purple shiso leaves (for serving)

Instructions:
1. Preheat the lower third of oven rack to 450 degrees F. Sprinkle with cornmeal over a baking sheet.
2. Roll out dough into a 12-inch oval on a lightly floured surface. Move to the prepared saucepan and brush with 1 spoonful of oil.
3. Sprinkle with garlic, 1/8 teaspoon salt and crushed red pepper, then mozzarella on top. Bake the dough for about 12 to 15 minutes, until golden brown and bubbling.

4. Meanwhile, pick off artichokes from the tough outer leaves and cut off the top two-thirds, down to the middle.
5. Peel the tough stem and remove any fuzzy choke by cutting the artichokes in half. Slice the artichokes thinly, and mix with lemon juice in a cup.
6. Using a vegetable peeler, peel asparagus into long strips; thinly slice what cannot be rasped.
7. Add the asparagus and pecorino, pepper, the remaining 1 tablespoon oil and 1/8 teaspoon salt into the bowl; mix to coat.
8. Put the vegetables on the pizza and sprinkle with zest of lemon and shiso, if required.

10) Stuffed Potatoes with Salsa Beans Salsa

With this basic recipe of loaded sweet potatoes with beans, salsa and avocados, Taco night means baked potato night. This balanced yet simple family dinner needs only 10 minutes active time so you can easily make it on the busiest weeknights too.

Active Time: 10-15 minutes| Total Time: 25-30 minutes| Servings: 4| Calories: 324 kcal

Ingredients:
- Russet potatoes: 4 mediums
- Fresh salsa: ½ cup
- Avocado: 1, sliced
- Pinto beans: 1 can (15 ounces), boiled and lightly mashed
- Pickled jalapeños: 4 teaspoons, chopped

Directions:
1. Pierce potatoes using a fork. Microwave for 20-22 minutes, turning the sides until moist.
2. Switch to a cutting board and allow them to cool.
3. Once cool cut the potatoes in cubes using a knife.
4. Top with avocado, beans, salsa and jalapenos on each potato. Serve!

11) Rice Black Bean Bowl with Tofu and Asparagus

Black beans and sesame seeds have potent antioxidant compounds which have been proven to minimize inflammation—eating these with black rice upgrades the nutrition. Simmer it in coconut milk to add rich flavor and aroma.

Active Time: 35 minutes| Total Time: 1 hour| Servings: 4| Calories: 577 kcal

Ingredients:
- Avocado oil: 3 tablespoons, divided
- Lemongrass: 1 tablespoon, chopped
- Garlic: 3 teaspoons, minced
- Black rice: 1 cup
- Coconut milk: 1 can (15 ounces)
- Water: ⅓ cup
- Salt: ¾ teaspoon, divided
- Sesame oil: 2 tablespoons toasted
- Tamari or soy sauce: 2 tablespoons, low-sodium

- Brown sugar: 1 tablespoon
- Red pepper: ¼ teaspoon crushed
- Extra-firm tofu: 1 package (14 ounces)
- Purple asparagus: 1 pound, trimmed and cut into 1-inch pieces
- Ginger: 1 tablespoon, grated
- Shredded coconut: ½ cup, unsweetened
- Lime juice: 1 tablespoon
- Black sesame seeds: 1 teaspoon
- 3 scallions, sliced
- For garnish: Thinly sliced purple daikon and basil leaves
- For serving: lime wedges

Directions:
1. Heat 1 tablespoon of avocado oil over low-medium heat in a saucepan. Add 1 tsp of garlic and lemongrass and cook, frequently stirring for around 30-35 seconds until fragrant. Add rice and mix. Add water, coconut milk and ½ tsp salt.
2. Simmer over high heat. Lower heat and cook for 35-45 minutes until the rice is soft and the water is absorbed.
3. Meanwhile, take a small bowl and mix tamari, sesame oil, brown sugar and red pepper. Cut the tofu into small cubes. Use paper towels to drain excess water.
4. Heat the rest 2 tbsps. of avocado oil over medium heat in a broad skillet. Add tofu in oil and cook, tossing once, for a minimum of 8-10 minutes until crispy and golden. Transfer to a dish and sprinkle 1/4 tsp of salt over it.
5. Add ginger, asparagus, and the remainder 2 tsp of garlic to the pan; cook, stirring, for about 3-4 minutes, until the asparagus is crispy and tender. Turn off heat. Whisk the sauce, then add the tofu to the sauce.
6. Add lime and coconut juice in rice.
7. Top the tofu mixture, scallions and sesame seeds over the rice. For serving use lime wedges and, where appropriate, garnish with daikon and basil.

12) Penne Pasta with Roasted Red Pepper and Spinach

This 20-minute penne pasta recipe is paired with roasted red peppers, garlic and spinach, and served with crumbled feta cheese for a quick and simple Mediterranean-style meal.

Active Time: 20 minutes| Total Time: 20 minutes| Servings: 6| Calories: 377 kcal

Ingredients:
- Whole-wheat penne: 12 ounces
- Garlic: 3 large cloves, diced
- Extra-virgin olive oil: ¼ cup
- Roasted red peppers: 1 jar (16 ounces), drained and chopped
- Baby spinach: 1 package (10 ounces)
- Salt: ½ teaspoon
- Ground pepper: ½ teaspoon
- Feta cheese: ¾ cup, crumbled

Directions:
1. Boil a half-filled saucepan of water, and cook pasta as instructed by the package. Drain water and return pasta to the pot.
2. In the meantime, heat oil over low-medium heat in a broad skillet. Add minced garlic and cook, frequently stirring, until fragrant.
3. Add spinach, roasted red peppers, salt and pepper and cook for about 4-5 minutes until the spinach is wilted.
4. Add pasta in the vegetable mixture. Top with crumbled feta cheese and serve.

13)   Vegan Udon Soup with Noodles

This noodles recipe in Japanese-style is packed with many Asian ingredients: miso, mirin (wine) and sesame oil.

Active Time: 35-40 minutes| Total Time: 40 minutes| Servings: 4| Calories: 325 kcal

Ingredients:
- Udon noodles: 4 ounces
- Canola oil: 1 tablespoon
- Fresh garlic: 1 ½ tablespoon, minced
- Fresh ginger: 1 tablespoon, grated
- Serrano pepper: 1
- Vegetable broth: 1 container (32 fluid ounce), low-sodium
- Mirin: 1 tablespoon
- Soy sauce: 1 tablespoon+ 1 teaspoon
- Cremini mushrooms: 2 cups, sliced
- Carrots: 1 cup, diced
- Baby bok choy: 2 heads, cut into 1-inch pieces
- Warm water: ½ cup
- White miso: 2 teaspoons
- Extra-firm tofu: 1 package (14 ounces), drained and cubed
- Scallions: ½ cup (4 medium), thinly sliced
- Sesame oil: 4 teaspoons, toasted, divided

Instructions:
1. Cook noodles as instructed in the package; drain water and put aside.
2. In the meantime, heat oil over low-medium heat in a broad pan. Add the ginger, garlic, and serrano; cook for about 1-2 minute, until fragrant.
3. Add mirin and broth and 1 tablespoon soy sauce and simmer. Add the carrots and mushrooms; simmer for 3-6 minutes, until the veggies are soft. Add bok choy and stir for 2 more minutes.
4. Whisk miso in warm until smooth and bring to the boil. Add tofu and cook for about 1-2 minute, until cooked through.
5. Add scallions in the broth.
6. Drizzle the soup over noodles. Sprinkle 1 teaspoon sesame oil and 1/4 teaspoon soy sauce and serve.

14)   Vegan Enchilada Casserole

Prep Time: 25-30 minutes| Total Time: 1 hour| Servings: 8| Calories: 357 kcal

Ingredients:
- Extra-virgin olive oil: 2 tablespoons
- Chopped onion: 1 cup
- Poblano peppers: ¾ cup, chopped
- Garlic: 6 cloves, minced
- Yellow squash: 1 medium, halved
- Zucchini: 1 medium, halved and sliced (1/4-inch)
- Fresh corn kernels: 1 cup
- Pico de gallo: 1 cup
- Salt: ½ teaspoon
- Pinto beans: 1 can (15 ounces), salt-free, rinsed
- Black beans: 1 can (15 ounces), salt-free, rinsed
- Corn tortillas: 8 (6 inches)
- Pepper Jack cheese: 1 ½ cups shredded
- Avocado: 1, diced
- Scallions: ½ cup
- Sour cream: ½ cup, low-fat

Instructions:
1. Set the oven to 350 F and preheat it. Heat the oil over low-moderate heat in a large skillet. Add the poblanos and garlic and cook for 4-5 minutes, frequently stirring, until softened.
2. Add cabbage, corn, zucchini, Pico de gallo and salt.
3. Cook for 5-7 minutes, occasionally stirring until the liquid decreases by half. Turn off the heat; stir in pinto beans and black beans.
4. Spray a 9/13-inch baking tray with almond oil. Spread 1/2 of the vegetable mixture onto the tray.
5. Put 4 tortillas over the mixture. Sprinkle the cheese over the tortillas evenly. Repeat the same procedure for the remaining vegetable mixture and tortillas.
6. Bake 25-30 minutes, until bubbles appear on cheese. Sprinkle with scallions and avocados, evenly.
7. Serve with sour cream.

15) Black Bean-Cauliflower "Rice" Bowl

This aromatic rice bowl of cauliflower is prepared in minutes and is a perfect dinner meal.

Active Time: 20-25 minutes| Total Time: 30 minutes| Servings: 1| Calories: 510 kcal

Ingredients:
- Olive oil: 1 tablespoon + 2 teaspoons, divided
- Cauliflower rice: 1 cup, frozen
- Salt: ⅛ teaspoon
- Chopped onion: 2 tablespoons
- Green bell pepper: 2 tablespoons, chopped
- Chilli powder: ½ teaspoon

- Ground cumin: ½ teaspoon
- Dried oregano: ¼ teaspoon
- Canned black beans: ⅔ cup, salt-free, rinsed
- Roasted red pepper: 2 tablespoons, chopped
- Water: ¼ cup
- Lime juice: 1 tablespoon
- Cheddar cheese: ¼ cup, low-fat, shredded
- Tomato: 1 medium, chopped
- Fresh cilantro: 1 tablespoon, chopped.

Instructions:
1. Heat 1 tablespoon of oil over low-moderate heat in a skillet. Add salt and cauliflower rice; cook for 3-5 minutes, frequently stirring, until cooked through.
2. Transfer to a dish.
3. In another skillet heat the remaining 2 teaspoons of oil over low-medium heat. Add green pepper, onion, chili powder, cumin and oregano; cook for about 3-4 minutes, frequently stirring, until the veggies are softened.
4. Add roasted red pepper, beans and the water; bring to a boil. Cook 3-5 minutes, frequently stirring, until cooked and thickened. Add lime juice after turning the heat off.
5. Layer the bean mixture into a dish with the soft cauliflower rice. Top with cheese and tomato. Use cilantro for garnishing, if you like.

16) Zucchini Noodle Primavera

This recipe cut out carbohydrates by replacing the zucchini noodles with pasta. This vegan dinner is packed with colorful veggies smothered in a sweet, creamy sauce.

Active Time: 15-20 minutes| Total Time: 25-30 minutes| Servings: 4| Calories: 313 kcal

Ingredients:
- Unsalted butter: 2 tablespoons
- All-purpose flour: 2 tablespoons (1 cup)
- Basil pesto: 3 tablespoons, refrigerated
- Extra-virgin olive oil: 1 tablespoon
- Cherry tomatoes: 2 cups, halved.
- Garlic: 4 cloves, sliced
- Salt: ¼ teaspoon
- Broccoli florets: 2 cups
- Red bell pepper: 1 cup thinly sliced
- Carrots: 1 cup, cut into matchsticks size
- Zucchini noodles: 2 packages (10 ounces), about 6 cups
- Parmesan cheese: ¼ cup, shredded
- Fresh basil: 2 tablespoons, chopped

Directions:
1. Melt the butter in a saucepan. Add flour gradually and keep on whisking until the mixture is thickened.

2. Add pesto; stir until well mixed. Turn off heat and rest aside.
3. Heat the oil over low-moderate heat in a broad skillet. Add garlic, tomatoes, and salt; cook, frequently stirring, for 3-4 minutes, until the garlic is fragrant and tomatoes turn into a paste.
4. Add bell pepper, broccoli, carrots and pesto mixture; cook for around 4-5 minutes until the broccoli is moist.
5. Add the noodles; gently shake to mix.
6. Cook for about 2-3 minutes, shaking gently until the noodles are well coated with the sauce.
7. Divide equally into 4 bowls; Serve with basil and parmesan.

17) Vegan "Pancit Bihon" with Spaghetti Squash

In this classic Filipino noodle recipe pancit bihon, shiitake mushrooms are used instead of beef, and spaghetti squash for conventional rice noodles. To make it a meal, serve with your preferred vegan main or cubed tofu.

Active Time: 20 minutes| Total Time: 1 hour| Servings: 4| Calories: 207 kcal

Ingredients:
- Spaghetti squash: 1 small, (1 3/4-2 pounds), seeds removed and halved.
- Coconut oil: 2 tablespoons
- Onion: 1 cup, chopped
- Garlic: 2 tablespoons minced
- Fresh ginger: 1 tablespoon, minced
- Shiitake mushroom caps: 2 cups sliced
- Green vegetables: 2 cups, shredded (e.g. cabbage, bok choy or kale)
- Carrot: 1 cup, shredded
- Salt: ¼ teaspoon
- Ground pepper: ¼ teaspoon
- Soy sauce: 1 tablespoon, low-sodium
- For serving: lemon wedges

Instructions:
1. Set the oven to 400 F and preheat.
2. Spread spaghetti squash, cut down in halves on a baking tray. Bake, for 35-40 minutes, until soft.
3. Once cool, remove the flesh from shells with the help of a fork.
4. Heat oil over low-medium heat in a broad skillet. Add garlic, onion and ginger, cook for 3-4 minutes until onions turn translucent. Add the mushrooms in it and cook for another 4-5 minutes, frequently stirring, until tender.
5. Add green veggies, salt and pepper and carrots; cook, stirring for 1-2 minutes until softened. Turn off the heat and stir soy sauce and spaghetti squash.
6. Garnish with lime wedges.

18) Vegan Gumbo

This vegan dinner is a classic Louisiana veggie version. It is chock-filled with tomatoes, butternut squash, poblano peppers and okra. This vegan gumbo is a fast dinner packed with flavor and spice and takes only 30 minutes active time.

Active Time: 30 minutes| Total Time: 30-35 minutes| Servings: 10| Calories: 322 kcal

Ingredients:
- All-purpose flour: ½ cup
- Extra-virgin olive oil: ⅓ cup
- Butternut squash: 1 small, cubed into 3/4- to 1-inch
- Yellow onions: 2 cups, chopped
- Poblano peppers: 2 cups, chopped
- Celery: 1 cup, chopped
- Vegetable broth: 8 cups, low-sodium
- Whole plum tomatoes: 1 can (28 ounces), drained and crushed
- Salt: 1 ¾ teaspoon
- Okra: 3 cups, trimmed and sliced
- Zucchini: 3 cups, chopped
- Pinto beans: 2 cans (15 ounces), rinsed.
- Hot sauce: 2 tablespoons
- Red-wine vinegar: 1 tablespoon
- Ground pepper: ½ teaspoon
- Brown rice: 4 cups, cooked

Instructions:
1. In a seven-quarter pot, whisk the oil and flour.
2. Cook over low-medium heat, occasionally stirring, until the mixture is dark brown, for 10-12 minutes.
3. Add cabbage, poblanos, onions, and celery; cook for about 5-6 minutes, frequently stirring, until the veggies are well coated and moist.
4. Add water, salt and crushed tomatoes; bring to a boil. Add okra; lower heat and simmer for 5-6 minutes.
5. Add the beans and zucchini; simmer for about 4-5 minutes, until the squash is tender. Garnish with chilli sauce, vinegar and seasoning. Serve with beans.

19) Noodles with Shiitakes, Bean Sprouts and Carrots

A Sriracha hit gives this balanced vegetarian recipe a spicy and sweet edge. Modern lo mein is made from fresh lo mein noodles, available in Asian markets. You may also use dried or fresh linguine noodles. This simple dinner is prepared in just 30-35 minutes, which makes it great for weekends.

Prep Time: 35 minutes| Total Time: 40 minutes| Servings: 4| Calories: 319 kcal

Ingredients:
- Fresh lo mein noodles: 8 ounces
- Sesame oil: 2 teaspoons, toasted
- Soy sauce: 3 tablespoons, Low-sodium
- Sriracha: 2 teaspoons

- Vegetable oil: 2 tablespoons, divided
- Minced garlic: 2 tablespoons
- Carrot: 1 large (about 1 cup), cut into half lengthwise and then cut 1/4-inch-thick half-moon shape slices
- Shiitake mushrooms: 4 ounces, stems removed and caps cut into 1/4-inch thick slices.
- Celery: 1 cup, thinly sliced
- Bean sprouts: 2 cups
- Fresh cilantro: 3 tablespoons, chopped

Instructions:
1. Bring water to boil in a half-filled pot.
2. Cook noodles as directed by box.
3. Drain the water. Move to a big bowl and sprinkle with sesame oil; rest aside.
4. In a tiny cup, mix Sriracha and soy sauce; rest aside.
5. Heat over low-medium heat a 12-inch stainless steel skillet. Add 1 tablespoon vegetable oil.
6. Add the garlic; stir-fry for about 10-12 seconds, until only fragrant. Add mushrooms, carrot and celery; stir-fry for about 1-2 minute until the celery turns bright green and the veggies have absorbed all the oil.
7. Stir in the remaining 1 tablespoon of oil. Add noodles, bean sprouts, and soy sauce; stir-fry for 1-2 minutes until the noodles are cooked through, and the veggies are crispy and tender. Add cilantro, toss and serve.

20) Spring Veggie Wraps

This veggie wrap recipe is a colorful mixture of tangy tahini-ginger-soy, both marinate the tofu and gives a spicy flavor. Go for spinach green tortillas for an extra pop.

Active Time: 25 minutes| Total: 1 hour 15 minutes| Servings: 4| Calories: 385 kcal

Ingredients:
- 1 (14 ounces) package extra-firm tofu, drained and cut into 1/4-inch-thick planks
- Tahini sauce: ¼ cup
- Orange juice: ¼ cup + 2 tablespoons, divided
- Lime juice: 1 tablespoon
- Soy sauce, low-sodium: 1 tablespoon
- Fresh ginger: 1 tablespoon, minced
- Garlic: 1 clove, minced
- Avocado or canola oil: 2 teaspoons divided
- Salt: ¼ teaspoon, divided
- Bibb lettuce: 8 large leaves
- Carrot: 1 cup, shredded
- Radishes: 6 mediums, thinly sliced
- Scallions, thinly sliced: 2 tablespoons
- Whole-wheat tortillas: 4 8-inch warmed

- Sesame seeds: 2 tablespoons

Instructions:
1. Use a paper towel, put tofu on it and press gently to drain excess water.
2. Move the tofu to a baking tray of 9/12-inch.
3. In a medium bowl, whisk together 1/4 cup orange juice, tahini, lime juice, ginger soy sauce, and garlic.
4. Save 1/4 cup of the mixture in the refrigerator for later use as a sauce. Add 2 tablespoons orange juice in the remaining mixture. Marinate the tofu in the mixture and refrigerate for 25-30 minutes.
5. Heat 1 teaspoon oil over low-medium heat in a broad skillet.
6. Add half the marinated tofu in oil and sprinkle 1/8 teaspoon salt; toss and cook for 4-6 minutes, until golden brown.
7. Place the tofu onto a dish and keep warm. Repeat the process with remaining tofu.
8. Arrange the carrots, lettuce, radishes, and scallions down the middle of each tortilla. Add the tofu, and pour the sauce you reserved over it. Serve with a sprinkle of sesame seeds.

2.5. Delicious Vegan Dessert Recipes

Such delicious vegan and dairy-free dessert recipes (from ice cream to no-bake brownies to the yummiest cheesecake) promise to satisfy every palate, whether you are a vegan, lactose intolerant or just craving anything sweet.

1) Strawberry Coconut Cream Pie

Prep Time: 10 mins| Total Time: 10 mins| Yield: 8-10

Ingredients:

For Pie Crust:
- Medjool dates: ¾ cup (about 11), soak in warm water for 5-6 minutes, then drain the water
- Raw cashews: 3/4 cup, chopped
- Unsweetened coconut: 1/4 cup, shredded

For Pie Filling:
- Coconut cream: 1 can (14-oz), refrigerate overnight
- Maple syrup: 2 tablespoons
- Vanilla extract: 2-3 drops
- Strawberries: 1 lb., sliced
- For Pie Topping:
- Toasted coconut
- Grated dark chocolate
- Fresh mint

Instructions:
1. Crust Preparation: Add cashew bits, drained dates, and coconut in a blender and blend until the mixture can be shaped into a ball easily.
2. Layer plastic wrap on an 8-inch round-shaped cake pan.

3. Dump the cashew-date-coconut mixture into the middle of the pan and flatten it with fingertips, gently pressing the sides of the pan. Put the pan freezer to set for a few minutes.
4. Filling preparation: Take the coconut milk out of the fridge. Scoop the solid white part out and put it in a hand mixer's bowl. Add the maple syrup, vanilla and whip for around 1-2 minutes until fluffy and smooth.
5. Assembling: Take the crust out from the freezer. Pour the filling over the crust, then use a spatula to smooth out the top. Put back in the freezer for 15-20 minutes.
6. After 10 minutes take out from the freezer and top with toasted coconut, strawberries, mint. Put back in the freezer for almost an hour.
7. Remove the pie gently from the pan and wrap. Cut and serve on a serving plate.

2) Almond Apricot Tart

Ingredients:
- Pie crust: 1 9-inch
- Apricot preserves: 1/4 cup
- Slivered almonds: 3/4 cup
- Apricots: 7-9
- Sugar: 1/3 cup
- Vegan butter: 1 tablespoon, cut into small cubes

Preparation:
1. Set the oven to 450 ° F and preheat. Roll the pie crust into around 10-11 inches and spread it gently onto the pie pan, pressing firmly on both the bottom and sides. Poke the bottom of the pastry using a fork, so it does not puff up during the process of baking.
2. Bake for 10-12 minutes or until crust turn golden brown.
3. When the pastry has been removed, raise the oven temperature to 375 ° F.
4. Add the almonds in a hand blender and blend until the almonds are chopped, but not crushed to powder. Put it aside.
5. Fill a large pot with water and ice of equal parts, set aside. - Bring a casserole of half-filled water to boil and add 2 to 3 apricots in it, simmer for 20-25 seconds and move to the ice bath for immediate cooling.
6. Repeat with the remaining apricots. Then peel and slice them in half using a sharp knife, removing the pits. Put on aside.
7. Layer the apricot jam in the base of the tart. Sprinkle with chopped almonds and make a second layer of apricot halves over the almonds, cut side down. Sprinkle with some sugar and bits of butter uniformly over the tart.
8. Bake for about 50-60 minutes, until apricots are soft.
9. Cool and serve!

3) Cherry Almond Cake

Calories: 425 kcal| Serves: 6| Cooking Time: 45 minutes
Ingredients:

- Spelt flour: 1 ¼ cup
- Almond flour: 1 ¼ cup
- Salt: 1/4 teaspoon
- Baking powder: 2 teaspoons
- Cinnamon: 1/2 teaspoons
- Coconut sugar: 1/2 cup
- Natural almond butter: 1/3 cup
- Maple syrup: 2 tablespoons
- Vanilla extract: 1/2 teaspoon (optional)
- Almond milk: 1 cup
- Cherries: 1 cup, frozen and pitted
- Slivered almonds

Preparation:
1. Set the oven to 320 °F and preheat.
2. Take a large bowl, and mix the first 6 ingredients, and stir to avoid any clumps.
3. Switch to the blender with maple syrup, almond butter, vanilla and oat milk. Blend all the ingredients.
4. Whisk the wet ingredients in a bowl. Then, fold the cherries in.
5. Move the dough to 7 inches of the lightly greased cake pan. Place a few cherries and slivered almonds on top, and gently press down.
6. Bake 45–50 minutes. Set aside to cool completely.
7. Garnish with coconut cream.

4) Skillet Strawberry S' mores

Active Time: 8-10 minutes| Cook Time: 10 minutes| Total Time: 18 minutes| Yield: 15 servings

Ingredients:
- Cast iron skillet: 8-inch
- Vegan butter: 1/2 tablespoon
- Vegan chocolate chips: 1 1/2 cups
- Vegan marshmallows: 15
- Vegan graham crackers

Instructions:
1. Put an 8-inch iron skillet into the oven's middle rack. Set the oven to 450 ° F and preheat it.
2. Once preheated, take the hot skillet out of the oven and put it on the stovetop. Coat the bottom of the pan with vegan butter. Layer the chocolate chips on the bottom of the pan, then layer the marshmallows over the chocolate chips in a way to completely cover the chocolate.
3. Put the skillet back in the oven for around 8-10 minutes, or until it on marshmallows turn light brown.
4. Serve with graham crackers right away.

5) Peach and Cream Cheesecake

A super easy and creamy summer cake! All vegan, gluten-free, refined sugar-free and no-bake.

Ingredients:
For the Filling:
- Cashews: 250 g, soak for 6 hours
- Maple syrup: 150 g
- Oat milk: 130 g
- Melted coconut oil: 110 g
- Lemon juice: 50 g
- Fresh peaches: 2
- Turmeric powder: 1 teaspoon
- Vanilla powder: 1/2 teaspoon
- Pinch of salt

For the Crust:
- White almonds: 200 g
- Shredded coconut: 25 g
- Pitted dates: 4

Instructions:
1. Note: The cashews can be soaked up to 24 hours before use. Only take a large tub, fill it up with the nuts and water. Bear in mind that the nuts suck up water and so leave some space for this.
2. Add the shredded coconut and almonds to your blender. Blend until you have a texture resembling flour.
3. Add the dates, and then blend again.
4. Take an 8-inch parchment paper cake pan and line with it. Press the crust into the saucepan uniformly, set aside.
5. Add the cashews with the oat milk, maple syrup, lemon juice, coconut oil, vanilla powder and salt and in the blender.
6. Fill a bowl with half the mixture. Put it aside.
7. Cut the peaches, remove the block, and add into the blender with turmeric powder.
8. Mix well and spread over the crust. Put in the freezer for 1 hour. Meanwhile, put the other bowl into your fridge with the filling.
9. Spread a second layer on the top of your peach layer and set in the freezer overnight.
10. Garnish with your choice of fresh fruits.

6) Lemon Custard
Serves: 6| Cooking Time: 5
Ingredients:
- Soy milk, unsweetened: 4 cups
- Cornstarch: 8 tablespoons
- Sugar: 6 tablespoons

- Turmeric: 2/8 teaspoon
- 1 lemon zest
- Vanilla extract: 1 teaspoon (optional)

Preparation:
1. Whisk the cornstarch, milk, sugar and turmeric together in a saucepan until well incorporated.
2. Place the saucepan over low-moderate heat and bring it to a simmer while continually whisking. Let the starch simmer gently for at least 1-2 minutes, frequently stirring to prevent any lumps, until desired consistency is achieved. Add the ingredients of flavoring (vanilla extract or lemon zest). If using lemon zest, make sure that only the yellow portion of the lemon is used, and not the white part under the skin.
3. Let the custard refrigerate at room temperature. Whisk occasionally to avoid skin formation on the surface. Let the pan in sit in cold water to cool down faster. Once cool serve!

7) Peanut Butter Chocolate Chip Cookie Bars

These cookies with peanut butter are my favorite treats for all time! They get a nice chocolate chip, peanut butter and a thick layer of cacao-date on top of it.

Serves: 25

Ingredients:
- Cookie Layer
- Creamy peanut butter: ½ cup + 2 tablespoons
- Melted coconut oil: ¼ cup + 1 tablespoon
- Maple syrup: ¼ cup + 1 tablespoon
- Vanilla extract: 2 teaspoons
- Heaping sea salt: ½ teaspoon
- Almond flour: 2 ½ cups
- Maca powder: 2 ½ tablespoons
- Chocolate chips: 1 cup
- Cacao Layer
- Walnuts: 1½ cups
- Cacao powder: 2 tablespoons
- Sea salt: ¼ teaspoon
- Medjool dates: 10, soft
- Water: 2 tablespoons
- For sprinkling on top: Flaky sea salt (optional)

Instructions:
1. Line parchment paper in an 8X8-inch baking pan. Stir the coconut oil, maple syrup, vanilla, peanut butter, and salt in a wide bowl, until mixed. Add maca and the almond flour and stir to blend until the mixture is thick.
2. Add the chocolate chips and fill into the pan. Put the pan in the freezer so it can firm up a little before creating the next coat.

3. Process the cacao powder, walnuts and sea salt in a food processor until the walnuts get well chopped. When the blade gets sticky, add the dates and pump to mix, add 2 tablespoons of water. Process until well combined, and then spread onto the layer of cookies. Where appropriate, sprinkle the sea salt.
4. Freeze it for 30-35 minutes (this will help them firm up and make cutting easier). Take out and slice into bars. Store the remaining bars into the fridge or freeze them. Let the bars thaw in at room temperature for around 13-15 minutes.

8) Chocolate Avocado Pudding Pops

Prep time: 9 hours 5 minutes| Total time: 9 hours 5 mins| Serves: 10 pops

This recipe of chocolate pudding is a great summer dessert! It is completely vegetarian because almond butter and avocado make the base smooth and creamy.

Ingredients:
- Ripe avocados: 2 mediums
- Chocolate chips: ¼ cup, melted
- Cocoa powder: 3 tablespoons
- Maple syrup: 3 tablespoons
- Almond butter: 3 tablespoons
- Vanilla extract: 1 teaspoon
- Almond milk Vanilla: 2 cups
- Sea salt: ¼ teaspoon

Topping:
- Chocolate chips: ½ cup
- Coconut oil: + ½ teaspoon
- Crushed nuts: pistachios or almonds

Instructions:
1. Add the avocados with the almond milk, maple syrup, cocoa powder, almond butter, cinnamon, sea salt and melted chocolate chips into a blender. Mix until smooth. Pour in the ice pop moulds and place in the freeze overnight, or for 9 hours or more.
2. Before removing, let the pops settle for a couple of minutes at room temperature and loose enough to pull out.
3. Additional topping: Mix the coconut oil and melted chocolate chips and drizzle on the pops, also sprinkle the nuts.
4. Instead, this can be eaten as pudding. Scoop into a blender or individual bowls after you combine the mixture, and chill in the refrigerator for at least 2-4 hours.

9) Best Vegan Ice Cream

Active Time: 20-25 minutes| Total time: 30 minutes| Serves: 4

This simple, milk-free ice cream is so delightful and rich! In this recipe, the tahini has no strong flavor; it just gives the base of coconut milk an extra-creamy texture.

Ingredients:

- Full-fat coconut milk: 1 can (14-ounce)
- Maple syrup: ⅓ cup
- Tahini: ¼ cup
- Toppings:
- Tart cherries
- Sesame seeds
- Chocolate

Instructions:
1. Refrigerate your Ice Cream Attachment frame for minimum 12 hours, ideally overnight.
2. Mix the maple syrup, tahini and coconut milk together in a wide cup. (If the coconut milk is chunky, you can put the ingredients together in a blender).
3. Pour the mixture into the ice cream machine, and churn for about 20 minutes until warm. Scoop out and have fun!
4. Freeze it for 1-2 hours, if you like thick texture.

Note:
If you have your ice cream stored in the refrigerator for more than 24 hours, it can harden. Set aside at room temperature to soften before scooping for 20 minutes.

10) Blackberry and White Chocolate Tart

Ingredients:
Crust:
- Oat flour: 1 cup
- Almond milk: 1 cup
- Maple syrup: 2-3 tablespoons (optional)
- Coconut oil: 1/4 cup
- Pinch of salt

For Filling:
- Cashews: 3/4 cup, soaked for 4-5 hours
- Fresh blackberries: 1 cup
- White chocolate (vegan): 200g
- Full-fat coconut milk: 2 cans
- Maple syrup: 1/4 cup
- Super color powder: 1/4 teaspoon
- Agar powder: 1 teaspoon

For Garnishing:
- Delaware grapes
- Fresh blackberries

Instructions:
Crust:
1. Set your oven at 180 Celsius. Oil an 8 inches tart plate. Set aside. Mix the crust ingredients into a food processor and mix well.

2. You must get a sticky mixture that can quickly be molded. Press tightly to the base and up the walls of the tart pan. Bake it for 25 mins until the crust becomes golden brown.
3. Move to a rack and let it cool while you prepare the filling.

Filling:
1. Place the saucepan over a low-medium heat and add the blackberries with 2 tablespoons of water. As it starts boiling mash the blackberries. Strain it and let them cool down. In a saucepan, add white chocolate and melt it then add coconut cream, and put at low heat. Add the maple syrup, agar-agar, and super color powder and make the mixture moist.
2. Stir it repeatedly, cook until the agar dissolves. Put the soaked cashew nuts, blackberry mixture, and the white chocolate-coconut cream into a food processor and blend.
3. Continue until smooth.
4. Fill the crust with this mixture. Place the tart overnight in the refrigerator to set. Garnish, and have fun!

11)   Coconut Mango Panna Cotta

Makes 4-6 depending Panna Cottas

Ingredients:

For the Panna Cotta:
- Coconut milk, unsweetened: 3 cups
- Maple syrup: 4 tablespoons
- Agar powder: 1 teaspoon
- Vanilla extract: ½ teaspoon

For the Jelly:
- Mango purée: 1 cup
- Maple syrup: 1 tablespoon (optional)
- Agar powder: ½ teaspoon
- For garnishing:
- Toasted coconut chips

Directions:

For the Panna Cotta:
1. Whisk all the ingredients together in a normal-sized pan over low-medium heat.
2. Boil the mixture and turn off the burner instantly. In 4-6 glasses or ramekins, equally, pour the mixture.
3. Let it refrigerate for 3-4 hours, until set.

For the Jelly:
1. In a medium-sized saucepan, over low-medium heat, whisk all the ingredients and bring it to boil.
2. Turn off the heat and allow for several minutes to cool down before pouring over. Transfer the panna cotta to the refrigerator for one hour to set the mango.
3. Before serving, toss the coconut chips on the top.

12) Frozen Yogurt Bars

An amazing homemade frozen Greek yoghurt bars with berries, or variations of your favorite fruit. Vegetarian and gluten-free, ideal for breakfast, a balanced meal!

Active Time: 10-15 minutes| Cook Time: 3 minutes| Freezing time: 4 hours| Total Time: 15 minutes| Servings: 10 people| Calories: 64kcal

Ingredients:
- Greek-style yogurt (Vegan): 2 cups
- Blueberries: 5 oz
- Fresh blackberries: 2 oz
- Vanilla extract: 1 teaspoon
- Juice of ½ lemon
- Maple syrup: 4 tablespoons

Instructions:
1. In a wide pan, add the blueberries and the lemon juice and bring it to a boil. Cook well until the blueberries have mixed up and let it cool.
2. Mix the Greek yogurt, maple syrup and vanilla in a medium dish. When cooled, add in blueberry sauce.
3. Layer a parchment paper in a baking dish and pour the yogurt mix in it.
4. Toss with some fresh blackberries, and freeze until solid for 4 to 5 hours. Slice them into bars of 2-3 inches, and enjoy.

13) Vegan Chocolate Pudding Recipe

Active time: 10-15 minutes| Cook time: 10 minutes| Chilling time: 4 hours| Yield: 4 to 8 servings

Ingredients:
- Full-fat coconut milk: 1 (15-ounce) can
- Dark chocolate (60-70%): 10 ounces, finely chopped
- Vanilla extract: 1 tablespoon, (optional)

For Garnishing:
- Shaved chocolate
- Whipped coconut cream
- Berries or other fresh fruit

Instructions:
1. Shake the coconut milk's can, before opening and pour into a small saucepan and warm it. Heat up coconut milk over low heat to a simmer. Stir in regularly to prevent scorching. Warm-up for a few minutes, until the liquid nearly boils. Remove it from heat immediately.
2. Add the chocolate:
3. Add 1/3 of the chopped chocolate in the hot coconut milk. Mix it gently until the chocolate has melted fully, and the paste is smooth. Continue in two different combinations, with the remaining chocolate. Whisk and add in the vanilla extract.

4. Take out the mixture into ramekins, glasses or jars. Wrap the plastic foil and place in the refrigerate for 4 hours.
5. To serve: Remove about 25 minutes before from the refrigerator. Top with your favorite toppings or simply serve with a spoon.

14) Vegan Mango Mousse

A Mousse, veggie-free, sugar-friendly and nice to taste! In this recipe, there is no gelatin or agar-agar, and it almost finished without additional sweetness.

Active Time: 12-15 minutes| Total Time: 1 hour| Servings: 4 people| Calories: 290 kcal

Ingredients:
- Mangoes: 3
- Coconut cream: 1 ½ cup
- Agave syrup: 3 tablespoons
- Powdered sugar: 2 tablespoons

Instructions:
1. Peel and slice the mangoes. Mash the slices to make a thick puree. Place the coconut cream in a large cup, and whisk the mango puree gently until it is smooth.
2. Add 3 tbsps of agave or sugar.
3. Season the Mousse with chocolate or shavings of fresh fruit.
4. This is it! Cool for 2-3 hours, and serve chilled!

15) Black and White Bombs

Ingredients:
- Slivered almonds: 2 cups
- Coconut oil: 1 cup
- Powdered sweetener: 1 - 2 tablespoon
- Vanilla extract: 2 teaspoons
- Orange zest: 1 teaspoon
- A pinch of kosher salt

Instructions:
1. Fill a small 12 cups muffin tray with small liners.
2. In a food processor, process the almonds oil, sweetener, zest and salt to a smooth mixture. Put the half mixture into a small bowl and add in powdered cocoa and whisk it.
3. Fill half of the muffin tray with the cocoa mixture and another half with vanilla. (You can have two colored cookies)
4. Repeat this process with the remaining mixture. Tap the tray on the table to prevent bubbles.
5. Freeze for about 25-30 minutes, until firm. Remove the liners if you want.
6. Put it in the fridge for max 4-5 days in an airtight jar.

16) Pineapple, Banana, Strawberry Skewers with Salted Chocolate Drizzle

Cook Time: 10 minutes| Prep Time: 15 minutes| Servings: 4 servings

Ingredients:
- Pineapple: 2 cups, cut into 1 1/2 -inch cubes
- Strawberries: 8
- Bananas: 2, sliced into 1 1/2-inch thick circles
- Coconut oil: 2 teaspoons
- Dark chocolate chips: 1/3 cup
- Coconut oil: 2 teaspoons
- Sea salt: 1/2 tsp
- Unsweetened coconut: 1/2 cup, toasted and shredded

Directions:
1. Use your skewers, to thread the pineapple pieces, bananas, and strawberries. Must soak in the water, when you use wooden skewers.
2. Heat the grill to low flame, put the fruits and brush with almond oil to avoid sticking.
3. Cook the skewers of fruits on the hot grill, for 2-3 minutes each side.
4. Turn off the grill and put the fruits on a tray. In a double boiler, make the chocolate dressing by heating up the coconut oil, choc chips and sea salt.
5. Keep swirling the chocolate till it is creamy, and then drizzle all over the fruits.
6. When you are not drizzling it on top, serve extra dipping with it.
7. Sprinkle with toasted chopped coconut, and voila!

17)   Mint Chocolate Chip Ice Cream

Prep Time: 15-10 minutes| Total Time: 4 hours, 15 minutes

Ingredients:
- Avocados: 2, peeled and pitted
- Full-fat coconut milk: 1 14 oz can
- Cashews: 1 cup
- Coconut oil: 1 tablespoon
- Medjool dates: 10
- Cacao nibs: 1/4 cup
- Mint leaves: 3/4 cup
- Vanilla extract: 1 tsp
- Sea salt: 1/4 tsp
- Liquid chlorophyll: 1 tablespoon (for color, optional)
- Chocolate Sauce Topping:
- Dark chocolate chips: 1/3 cup
- Coconut oil: 1 teaspoon

Directions:
1. For 2-3 hours, put the coconut milk in the freezer or overnight in the refrigerator.
2. In warm water, soak the cashews for at least 2 hours, and the dates for 15 mins.

3. Once you have cooled the coconut milk, open the can and take out the tough cream from the top and put it into your food processor. You can reserve the liquid, make smoothies by using it.
4. Drain the dates and cashews, and put them with all ingredients to the blender except the cacao nibs. While it is blending, use it to move the ingredients towards the blade when your blender comes with a plunger.
5. Or just keep stopping, scrape down the sides and blend. It will take approximately 5 mins.
6. Into a loaf pan lined with parchment, pour the ice cream, using a silicone spatula, make sure you get everything out of the blender.
7. Blend the cacao nibs until well blended.
8. Use plastic foil to cover the pan and freeze for 4-5 hours or until you are ready to eat.
9. Make homemade melted chocolate in a double boiler, by melting chocolate chips and spoon in coconut oil until silky; drizzle them directly over ice cream.

18) Vegan Blueberry Muffins

Active Time: 15-20 Minutes| Total Time: 40-45 Minutes| Serves: 12

Ingredients:
- Cooking spray
- All-purpose flour: 2 cups
- Baking powder: 2 teaspoons
- Kosher salt: ½ teaspoon
- Brown sugar: ⅔ cup
- Soy milk yogurt: ½ cup
- Almond milk, unsweetened: ⅓ cup
- Vegetable oil: ⅓ cup
- Applesauce, unsweetened: ¼ cup
- Vanilla extract: 1 teaspoon
- Blueberries: 2 cups
- Turbinado sugar: 2 tablespoons

Instructions:
1. Set your oven at 350ºF. Fill a 12-muffin baking tray with paper liners, and brush with cooking spray.
2. In a wide bowl, whisk together the baking powder, flour and salt. In another medium bowl, whisk the yogurt, vanilla, almond milk, brown sugar, butter and applesauce together.
3. With a spatula, gently mix the dry and wet mixture. Shortly before the batter gets thoroughly combined, mix in the blueberries. Equally, divide the batter among the muffin tray. Sprinkle the turbinado sugar on the muffin tops—Bake for 20-24 mins and test by inserting a knife in the center until it comes out clean. Let the tray cool for a couple of minutes, then remove and place on a rack.

19) Peanut Butter Cups

Makes: 12

Ingredients:
Vegan chocolate chips: 1 bag (approximately 1 1/2 cups)
Peanut butter: 1/4 cup

Directions:
1. Place a paper liner in a muffin tray or use a silicone muffin tray
2. Then melt the chocolate chips in a boiler until its smooth. On the bottom of the muffin liners, put 1 tablespoon of melted chocolate and spread it evenly with a spatula. Let it sit in the fridge for 10-15 minutes.
3. Then put 1 tablespoon of peanut butter on top of the chocolate which is hardened. Do not spread this out with your finger as it settles down and mostly remains in the middle. Refrigerate for 10 minutes.
4. When your chocolate has become sludger, just put it back in the double boiler to re-melt it quickly. Now take 1 or 2 more teaspoons of melted chocolate and bring it over the peanut butter. The peanut butter is not going to be super hard, but it is going to hold up for the remaining process.
5. Using your knife, you could even spread the melted chocolate a little in the sides to make sure it runs down to cover the peanut. It will not happen, particularly if the peanut butter portion is not refrigerated.
6. If you want, smooth the top of the cups, but they might just settle comfortably on their own. So, cool it down for at least 15-20 minutes before serving. If you want softer cups, place them in the refrigerator in an airtight jar or at room temperature.

20) Cocoa Silken Pudding

Active Time: 5 Minutes| Total Time: 5-10 Minutes| Serves: 1

Ingredients:
- Silken tofu: 1 block (19 oz)
- Raw cacao powder: ¼ cup
- Maple syrup: 3 - 4 tablespoon
- Almond milk: 1 tablespoon
- Sea salt: a pinch

Instructions:
1. Blend all the ingredients in a hand blender until smooth and creamy.
2. When you use cocoa powder, it tastes very bitter, so just put 1 tbsp of maple syrup or honey to make it taste sweeter.
3. For the extra sweet and salty combination, sprinkle a pinch of sea salt over the top, when serving the pudding.

Part 3: 7 Day Sample Meal Plans

This part covers sample meal plans covering the whole week of vegan meals to help you begin with the vegan diet and improving your strength and endurance.

Chapter 3: Sample Meal Plans to increase Strength and Endurance

Vegans may be at elevated risk for deficiencies of other nutrients. A well-planned vegan diet that contains fortified nutrient-rich foods will help to provide a sufficient level of nutrients. Here are 2 sample meal plans mentioned below for vegan athletes.

Meal plan 1 is a high-carb, low-fat plan with a 50% carb, 25% fat and 25% protein macronutrient ratios that will help you boost your strength.

Meal plan 2 is a low-carb, high-fat plan with a 30% carb, 45% fat and 25% protein macronutrient ratios, perfect for increasing stamina.

Both meal plans contain a significant amount of protein that is 25% of the total calories. Whether you are eating a diet higher or lower in carbs depends on:
- Your skin
- The goals
- Your genetic makeup
- The sport and level of operation

No one can tell how to eat, so you are not expected to adjust what to eat based on what works for someone. It may take some research to find it out. However, most people do better with a moderate intake of about 50% carbs, with the majority of their calories coming from proteins and fats.

3.1. Vegan Sample Meal Plan for Increasing Strength

A high-carb and low-fat meal plan to give your strength a boost!

Monday
- Breakfast: Tofu scramble and a plant-milk chai latte.
- Snacks: Fruit and nut butter
- Lunch: Tofu Tacos and vegetarian kale Caesar salad.
- Dinner: Roasted veggie brown rice bowl.

Tuesday
- Breakfast: Overnight oats with fruits on the bottom, fortified plant milk, chia seeds and nuts.
- Snacks: Guacamole and crackers
- Lunch: Edamame hummus wraps.
- Dinner: Thai peanut curry noodles.

Wednesday
- Breakfast: A glass of mango and spinach smoothie and an easy baked oatmeal muffin.
- Snacks: Roasted Chickpeas
- Lunch: Stuffed potatoes with salsa and beans.
- Dinner: Black bean cauliflower rice bowl.

Thursday
- Breakfast: Whole-grain toast with banana, hazelnut butter and a fortified plant yogurt.

- Snacks: Edamame with sea salt
- Lunch: Cabbage lentil soup.
- Dinner: Eggplant Lasagna.

Friday
- Breakfast: Chocolate chip oatmeal cookie pancakes and a cappuccino made with fortified plant milk.
- Snacks: Hummus and Veggies.
- Lunch: Spring veggie wraps.
- Dinner: Vegan black bean burgers.

Saturday
- Breakfast: Avocado-Tofu toast and a glass of simple strawberry smoothie.
- Snacks: Rice cakes and avocado.
- Lunch: Roasted red pepper and ginger soup with whole-grain toast and hummus.
- Dinner: Roasted veggie brown rice bowl.

Sunday
- Breakfast: Sweet potato bowl and a glass of fortified orange juice.
- Snacks: Fruit and nut bars
- Lunch: Vegetarian lettuce wraps with a side of sautéed mustard greens.
- Dinner: Zucchini noodles primavera.

Remember to vary your carbs and protein sources during the day, as each provides various vitamins and minerals which are important for good health.

3.2 . Vegan Sample Meal Plan for Increasing Endurance

A low-carb and high-fat meal plan to boost your stamina!

Monday
- Breakfast: Jelly chia pudding with peanut butter with a glass of strawberry smoothie.
- Snacks: Strawberry rolls with a bowl of oatmeal.
- Lunch: Black bean chili with sweet potato and avocado salad.
- Dinner: Soybeans hummus wraps.

Tuesday
- Breakfast: Mushroom bacon toast with hummus and a glass of spinach, mango and banana Juice.
- Snacks: 2 nutty fruit bars.
- Lunch: Thai curry noodles with peanuts.
- Dinner: Vegan soup with noodles.

Wednesday
- Breakfast: A glass of carrot mango, spinach smoothie with burritos filled with tofu.
- Snacks: A banana with 1 or 2 tablespoons of raw cashew butter.
- Lunch: Stuffed potatoes with salsa beans and spring vegetable salad.
- Dinner: Vegetarian lettuce wraps.

Thursday
- Breakfast: Tater tot waffles and a grapefruit mango smoothie.
- Snacks: Cocoa strawberry balls with vegan protein pancakes.
- Lunch: Purple artichoke pizza with asparagus.
- Dinner: Black bean-cauliflower rice bowl.

Friday
- Breakfast: Black bean and sweet potato burritos with a glass of carrot, spinach and ginger juice.
- Snacks: A bowl of berries with some yogurt and rice cakes with avocado.
- Lunch: Mexican salad with tortilla croutons.
- Dinner: Zucchini noodle primavera.

Saturday
- Breakfast: A glass of gazpacho delight with chocolate chip and oatmeal pancakes.

Snacks: hummus with veggies, 1 orange or raw seeds and nuts.
- Lunch: Spinach and apple salad.
- Dinner: Penne pasta with spinach and roasted red pepper.

Sunday
- Breakfast: Cinnamon butter fig toasts with mango carrot and banana basil smoothie.
- Snacks: salsa with tortilla chips, 1 green apple and 2 tablespoons of raw almond butter
- Lunch: Tomato and rice soup with chickpeas.
- Dinner: Noodles with shiitakes, bean sprouts and carrots.

Conclusion

Athletes following a vegan diet or contemplating a vegan diet should pay careful attention to what they are consuming. Be sure to select nutrient-dense foods from the 100 delicious recipes listed above that include carbohydrate, protein and fat with enough nutrition, plus the minerals and vitamins needed to help oxygen delivery, recovery and immunity. Choose nutritious meals and snacks to fuel you without any gastrointestinal discomfort, before and after exercise. After your workouts, your food choices will help recovery too. It is crucial for all athletes, but particularly for vegans, to choose the right meals/snacks after practice.

If you are following a vegan diet, check the sample meal plans and make sure you are selecting the right meals. If you need help, ask a sports dietitian for advice.

CPSIA information can be obtained
at www.ICGtesting.com
Printed in the USA
LVHW060620200221
679377LV00007B/203